The Functional Foodie

50 Powerhouse Ingredients Go Gourmet

Ayn Nix and Andi Phillips

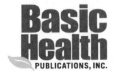

Basic Health
PUBLICATIONS, INC.

The information contained in this book is based upon the research and personal and pro-fessional experiences of the authors. It is not intended as a substitute for consulting with your physician or other healthcare provider. Any attempt to diagnose and treat an illness should be done under the direction of a healthcare professional. The ingredients featured in this book are not intended to be used as a treatment for any disease.

The publisher does not advocate the use of any particular healthcare protocol but believes the information in this book should be available to the public. The publisher and authors are not responsible for any adverse effects or consequences resulting from the use of the suggestions, preparations, or procedures discussed in this book. Should the reader have any questions concerning the appropriateness of any procedures or preparation mentioned, the authors and the publisher strongly suggest consulting a professional healthcare advisor.

Basic Health Publications, Inc.
28812 Top of the World Drive
Laguna Beach, CA 92651
949-715-7327 • www.basichealthpub.com

Library of Congress Cataloging-in-Publication Data

Nix, Ayn
    The functional foodie : 50 powerhouse ingredients go gourmet / text by Ayn Nix ;
recipes by Andi Phillips.
        p. cm.
    Includes bibliographical references and index.
    ISBN 978-1-59120-265-3
    1. Functional foods. I. Phillips, Andi. II. Title.
    QP144.F85N59   2010
    613.2—dc22

                                                                    2010030871

Editor: Cheryl Hirsch
Book design: Gary A. Rosenberg
Cover design: Mike Stromberg
Color photos: John Kelly • Black & white photos: Michael Sikov
Food styling, color photos: Liesl Maggiore
Cover art: Shutterstock

Printed in the United States of America

10   9   8   7   6   5   4   3   2   1

Contents

Introduction, 00

And now a word about my mom and dad . . .
I love you.

—ANDI PHILLIPS

Introduction

THERE IS A PERVASIVE BELIEF AMONG FOODIES and health nuts alike that eating healthfully means bravely stomaching wheat grass smoothies and suffering through bland plates of tasteless offerings possibly resembling Styrofoam. In other words, it's an either/or proposition: eat healthfully and give up much of your enjoyment of food, or live the good life of sumptuous sauces, rich desserts, wine and the like (and possibly develop a bad case of gout or worse). This book will put an end to this way of thinking once and for all! These recipes feature fifty of the hottest functional foods and ingredients—all backed by research for their health-promoting benefits. Powerful phytochemicals that have shown promise to fight cancer, nutritional compounds that can lower blood pressure, anti-aging antioxidants that protect against free-radical damage, and much more can all be found within the pages of this book—and in these recipes, they are surprisingly delicious.

These dishes can be confidently served at a dinner party attended by your most discriminating foodie friends, or simply made part of an everyday plan to eat well. But they should not be thought of as part of any kind of "diet." Rather, they are a way to take the best that nature has to offer and eat well—in every sense of the word. The bottom line is, these foods have medicinal properties, and maximizing their consumption every day can make you healthier. The ingredients have been chosen to maximize the nutritional potential and flavor of the dishes, and we want people to understand that they don't have to go on some crazy eating plan in order to weave these phytochemical-rich, antioxidant-rich, heart-healthy foods into their diet.

Many functional foods are "ordinary," everyday foods that science is discovering have some miraculous powers. Some are trendy new finds that many people are stumped by when it comes to how to prepare or enjoy. Some may surprise you—for example, in this book, chocolate is on a par with asparagus, and coffee is a health drink! In any case, you'll find delicious recipes, plus easy tips to try when you don't feel like cooking. Each recipe features a star ingredient and supporting ingredients that are wholesome and unprocessed. Most of the featured ingredients appear in more than one recipe, so flip through and try what you like. We sincerely hope you enjoy every bite.

Ayn Nix and Andi Phillips
(a.k.a. The Functional Foodies)

1. AGAVE NECTAR

Native Americans believed agave nectar could purify the body and soul. While we can't promise this, we certainly believe it can do the body and soul some good—especially in this heavenly Cranberry-Chocolate Tart recipe. This natural sweetener is derived from the agave cactus, which thrives in the volcanic soils of southern Mexico and is also used to make tequila. Agave nectar (sometimes called agave syrup) is sweeter than honey and table sugar, but is much lower on the glycemic index. This means agave doesn't stimulate digestive insulin secretion the way sugar does, which makes it a good sweetener choice even for diabetics. Agave also contains a beneficial fructan called inulin, and saponins, a type of phytochemical found in many plants, fruits, and vegetables that has been shown to have medicinal properties.

HEALTH BENEFITS

Research shows compounds and nutrients found in agave may benefit:

Chronic fatigue syndrome (CFS): Magnesium is needed for the synthesis of adenosine triphosphate (ATP, a primary energy source for cells), and is often low in CFS sufferers.

Colorectal cancer: Saponins may slow growth of tumors and are associated with a reduced risk.

Constipation: Inulin acts as a natural laxative.

Digestive health: Inulin promotes gastrointestinal health by acting as a prebiotic (food) for probiotics—beneficial bacteria that help with digestion.

High cholesterol and triglycerides: Inulin appears to lower elevated cholesterol and triglyceride levels.

Immunity: Inulin shows promise in fighting infection.

Liver disease: Fructans have been found to lower triglycerides in the liver.

Osteoporosis: One ounce supplies 12 percent of the Daily Value of calcium, necessary for maintaining strong bones; inulin is also associated with bone health and possibly helps by increasing calcium absorption.

Type 2 diabetes: Agave is low-glycemic, so it won't spike blood sugar.

Weight control and weight loss: Saponins reduce absorption of fat in the intestines, and fructans may promote weight loss (see Health Spotlight).

Wound healing: Agave contains antibacterial and anti-inflammatory compounds, which explains why ancient Aztecs used the sap topically, often mixed with salt, to treat wounds.

AGAVE NECTAR NUTRITION INFORMATION

Serving Size 1 ounce agave nectar (about 1 tablespoon)

Amount Per Serving

Calories 19	Calories from fat 0

	% Daily Value*
Total Fat 0 grams	0%
Saturated fat 0 gm	0%
Trans fat 0 gm	†
Cholesterol 0 milligrams	0%
Sodium 0 mg	0%
Total Carbohydrate 5 gm	2%
Dietary fiber 2 gm	7%
Sugars 1 gm	†
Protein 0 gm	0%
Vitamin A	0%
Vitamin C	2%
Calcium	12%
Iron	3%
Also contains:	
Magnesium	4%
Copper	2%
Vitamin K	2%
Manganese	1%

Agave's glycemic index (GI) ranking is only 27. In comparison, glucose has a GI of 100.

† Daily Value not established.

* Percent Daily Values are based on a 2,000-calorie diet.

HEALTH SPOTLIGHT

Double Duty for Diabetics

Diabetics not only benefit from agave's lower sugar content but also from its fructan content. Obesity and type 2 diabetes are linked to modifications of fatty acid metabolism, leading to the accumulation of triglycerides in the liver. In a study published in the *Journal of Nutrition*, consumption of fructans was shown to promote weight loss and lower triglycerides in the liver.

QUICK TIPS

❖ As a general rule, substitute $^3/_4$ cup of agave syrup for every cup of sugar in recipes.

❖ Agave dissolves easily in hot and cold drinks. Try it in smoothies and coffee, or on oatmeal.

Cranberry-Chocolate Tart

YIELD: 12 SERVINGS

Chocolate Short Crust
1 cup (2 sticks) unsalted organic butter
$^1/_2$ cup xylitol*
1 teaspoon vanilla extract
$^1/_2$ cup organic cocoa powder
$1^1/_2$ cups whole-wheat flour

Cranberry Filling
10 ounces frozen cranberries
$^1/_2$ cup fresh squeezed orange juice (about 2 oranges)
$1^1/_4$ cups agave syrup
1 vanilla bean, split lengthwise
Zest from squeezed oranges (zest before juicing)

Ganache Filling
5 ounces unsweetened chocolate, finely chopped
4 ounces cream cheese, at room temperature

5

$^1/_2$ cup agave syrup

$^1/_2$ cup soymilk

Special Equipment

12-inch tart pan with removable bottom

Parchment paper

Pie weights

*Xylitol, also called *birch sugar,* is available in most markets. It is a sugar alcohol found in the bark of birch trees and in the fibers of fruits and vegetables, including raspberries, corn husks, oats, and mushrooms. It looks and tastes like sugar, but has a low glycemic index so it is ideal for diabetics. It does not cause tooth decay, and studies show it may even repair minor cavities, as well as benefit osteoporosis by promoting calcium absorption.

TO MAKE THE DOUGH: In the bowl of a stand mixer, cream the butter, xylitol, and vanilla until smooth. Stop the mixer and scrape down the sides of the bowl. Add the cocoa powder and flour. Mix the dough just enough to combine. It should be evenly brown and have a grainy appearance. Press the dough into the bottom and up the sides of a 12-inch tart pan. Refrigerate the dough until it is firm, about 1 hour. Preheat oven to 350°F.

TO MAKE THE FILLING: While the dough is chilling, make the cranberry filling. In a medium-sized saucepan combine the cranberries, orange juice, agave syrup, and vanilla bean. Simmer the mixture over medium-low heat, stirring frequently until the filling is jam-like in consistency— about 30 to 40 minutes. Remove the vanilla bean and stir in orange zest. Allow the mixture to cool.

Gently press the parchment paper onto the surface of the tart crust. Fill the shell with pie weights, and bake it at 350°F on the center rack of the oven for 30 minutes. Place the pastry shell on a wire cooling rack. Once it has cooled, remove the pie weights and parchment paper. Spread the cranberry mixture over the bottom of the pastry shell. Set aside.

TO MAKE THE GANACHE: Place the finely chopped chocolate in a heat-proof bowl. In the bowl of a stand mixer, beat the cream cheese until smooth. While the mixer is running slowly add the agave syrup, then the soymilk in a thin stream. Beat the cream cheese mixture until smooth. Transfer the mixture to a small saucepan. Heat the mixture, stirring constantly, just until you see small bubbles come to the surface. Pour the hot cream cheese mixture over chocolate. Stir vigorously until you have a smooth glossy ganache. Pour the ganache over the cranberry layer and refrigerate until the ganache is firm. Remove the tart from pan and serve.

*   *   *

For other recipes and ways of using agave nectar, see: Banana Quick Tips (page 41), Banana Upside-Down Breakfast Cake (page 41), Blueberry Quick Tips (page 55), Blueberry Quick Bread (page 56), Goji Berry Granola (page 107), Millet Quick Tips (page 128), Pumpkin Oatmeal (page 137), Quinoa Quick Tips (page 168), Truffles (page 91), Watermelon Quick Tips (page 216), Watermelon Chiller (page 216), Yogurt Quick Tips (page 220), Yogurt with Chocolate-Peanut Butter Muesli (page 220).

2. ALMONDS

Go a little nuts! Almonds are a rich source of fiber, protein, vitamin E, manganese, magnesium, and copper and contain numerous flavonoids, especially in their skin. One study showed that the flavonoids in the skin of almonds plus the vitamin E content in the nut work together to have a favorable effect on low-density lipoprotein (LDL), or "bad," cholesterol. And even though almonds are a high-fat food, many studies show the monounsaturated fats found in almonds help lower cholesterol considerably. In fact, research published in the *American Journal of Clinical Nutrition* showed almonds contributed to a diet that lowered cholesterol as much as some statin drugs!

HEALTH BENEFITS

Research shows compounds and nutrients found in almonds may benefit:

Cataracts: Vitamin E helps protect the eye lens from damage by free radicals and lower risk of cataracts.

Digestive health: Fiber improves digestion and is linked to a reduced risk of hemorrhoids and diverticulitis (bulging tissue pouches in the colon).

Fatigue: Manganese works synergistically with copper and riboflavin to boost energy.

Gallstones: One ounce of nuts a week may reduce risk by 25 percent.

Heart health: Magnesium improves blood flow in arteries and helps maintain proper heart function.

High cholesterol: Monounsaturated fats appear to reduce LDL (bad) cholesterol, plus antioxidants may keep LDL cholesterol from oxidizing and damaging arteries.

Inflammation: Almonds have been shown to lower C-reactive protein (CRP, a marker indicating inflammation in the arteries).

Migraine headache: Magnesium relaxes muscles and nerves and is often low in migraine sufferers.

Osteoporosis: Calcium and manganese help keep bones strong.

Reproductive health: Manganese activates key enzymes responsible for production of sex hormones.

Skin health: Antioxidants and monounsaturated fats work to promote youthful skin.

Thyroid health: Manganese is required for normal thyroid function (the gland that helps to regulate body temperature and metabolism).

Type 2 diabetes: Eating nuts can reduce blood sugar after meals.

Weight control and weight loss: Fiber and monounsaturated fats promote satiety (see Health Spotlight).

ALMONDS NUTRITION INFORMATION

Serving Size 1 ounce almonds (about 25)

Amount Per Serving

Calories 170	Calories from fat 130

	% Daily Value*
Total Fat 15 grams	23%
Saturated fat 1 gm	5%
Trans fat 0 gm	†
Cholesterol 0 milligrams	0%
Sodium 0 mg	0%
Total Carbohydrate 5 gm	2%
Dietary fiber 4 gm	16%
Sugars 1 gm	†
Protein 7 gm	14%
Vitamin A	0%
Vitamin C	0%
Calcium	8%
Iron	6%
Also contains:	
Manganese	35%
Vitamin E	30%
Magnesium	20%
Potassium	6%

† Daily Value not established.
* Percent Daily Values are based on a 2,000-calorie diet.

HEALTH SPOTLIGHT

Prevent Weight Gain

Sounds almost too good to be true, but eating high-fat nuts can actually prevent you from gaining weight. In a study published in *Obesity*, people who ate nuts twice per week had a reduced risk of gaining weight compared to people who did not eat nuts. Over the course of the more than two-year study, those who enjoyed nuts were 31 percent less likely to gain weight than their counterparts who did not eat nuts and gained weight. It's probable that the fat and fiber provides satiety that prevents less-healthy snacking.

QUICK TIPS

❖ Divide almonds into small sandwich bags (about 25 per bag) to be stashed in your car, purse, and gym bag for snack emergencies. This serving size contains about the same number of calories as the average energy bar without the hydrogenated oils and sugars of some bars.

❖ Sprinkle chopped or slivered almonds on cereal, yogurt, and salads.

Scallops in Almond-Herb Sauce

YIELD: 4 SERVINGS

Almond-Herb Sauce

1 cup almond meal

1 scallion, green and white parts, roughly chopped

1 small fresh Thai chili pepper, halved, seeds removed

$1/4$ cup basil leaves

$1/4$ cup mint leaves

$1/4$ cup cilantro leaves

2 teaspoons finely grated ginger

2 cloves garlic, crushed

$1/2$ teaspoon lime zest (zest before juicing)

2 tablespoons fish sauce

1 tablespoon lime juice

$1/2$ cup almond milk

Scallops

1 pound bay scallops

2 tablespoons grape seed oil

8 ounces buckwheat noodles

Have all the ingredients measured and prepared before you begin to cook pasta.

TO MAKE THE SAUCE: As pasta cooks, in the bowl of a food processor combine the almond meal, scallion, chili, basil, mint, cilantro, ginger, garlic, zest, fish sauce, and lime juice. With the processor running, pour in the almond milk in one thin stream. Continue to process until it is a smooth sauce.

TO COOK THE SEAFOOD: Pat the scallops dry with a clean towel. Heat the oil on high in a large skillet. Add the scallops. Cook, turning the scallops constantly, about 2 minutes. Remove skillet from heat. Drain the pasta and return it to the cooking pot. While the pasta is still hot add the scallops (with any liquid that may be in the pan) and the sauce. Toss to coat everything. Serve immediately.

* * *

For other recipes and ways of using almonds, see: Apple-Almond Pilaf (page 19), Date Quick Tips (page 96), Whole-Wheat Maple Schmootz Muffins (page 119), Smoky Sweet Potatoes (page 200).

3. ANCHOVIES

As a pizza topping, anchovies may not be the most popular, but they definitely beat pepperoni when it comes to health benefits. These small silver fish are packed with heart-healthy omega-3 fatty acids; the B vitamins riboflavin (B_2), niacin (vitamin B_3), and cobalamin (vitaminB_{12}); and the minerals calcium and selenium. Canned anchovies, anchovy paste, and anchovy oil are common in Italian cooking, adding authentic Italian flavor as well as nutrition to many recipes. Anchovies lend a richer, saltier flavor to recipes without a fishy taste, so many people like them even if they are not fans of seafood (and probably don't even know they are eating them in their favorite Italian dishes). Keep in mind that anchovies are high in sodium—one 2-ounce can contains nearly 70 percent of your Daily Value of sodium—so enjoy them in moderation as the Italians do.

HEALTH BENEFITS

Research shows compounds and nutrients found in anchovies may benefit:

Alzheimer's disease: Docosahexaenoic acid (DHA), an omega-3 fatty acid, helps destroy Alzheimer's plaques in the brain; a high intake of niacin-rich foods may lower Alzheimer's risk by up to 70 percent.

Bipolar disorder: Eating a diet rich in seafood may be effective in reducing risk of bipolar disorder.

Cancer (blood or bone marrow, esophageal, kidney, mouth, pancreatic, stomach, and skin cancers): Selenium helps break down toxic chemicals and stimulates the immune system to fight cancer cells; DHA has been found to reduce tumor size.

Cataracts: Riboflavin may protect against formation of cataracts.

Colon cancer: Regular consumption of omega-3-containing foods has been shown to reduce risk by up to 37 percent; riboflavin may prevent colon polyps from becoming cancerous.

Dementia: Diets high in omega-3s may prevent cognitive decline in older adults.

Dry-eye syndrome: Omega-3s help alleviate this condition, in which decreased tear production fails to adequately lubricate the eye's surface .

Heart arrhythmia: Omega-3s are thought to stabilize heartbeat.

Heart attack: Omega-3s may reduce the risk of heart rhythm problems; niacin and vitamin B_{12} inhibit the buildup of homocysteine (a potentially toxic chemical and significant risk factor for heart disease).

High blood pressure: Diets high in omega-3 foods are associated with lower blood pressure; niacin also lowers high blood pressure.

High cholesterol: Omega-3s increase HDL (good) cholesterol; niacin decreases LDL (bad) cholesterol and increases blood flow.

ANCHOVIES NUTRITION INFORMATION

Serving Size 1 can anchovies (2 ounces)

Amount Per Serving

Calories 94	Calories from fat 39

	% Daily Value*
Total Fat 4 grams	7%
Saturated fat 1 gm	5%
Trans fat 0 gm	†
Cholesterol 38 milligrams	13%
Sodium 1,650 mg	69%
Total Carbohydrate 0 gm	0%
Dietary fiber 0 gm	0%
Sugars 0 gm	†
Protein 13 gm	21%
Vitamin A	0%
Vitamin C	2%
Calcium	10%
Iron	12%
Also contains:	
Omega-3 fatty acids 597 mg	†
Vitamin B_3 (niacin)	45%
Selenium	44%
Vitamin B_2 (riboflavin)	10%
Vitamin B_{12} (cobalamin)	7%

† Daily Value not established.
* Percent Daily Values are based on a 2,000-calorie diet.

Hyperactivity: Children taking omega-3 supplements showed significant improvement in symptoms of ADHD.

Immunity: Selenium protects the immune system, possibly by preventing the formation of free radicals and aiding in the production of antibodies.

Obesity: Eicosapentaenoic acid (EPA), an omega-3 fatty acid, stimulates the secretion of leptin, a hormone that helps regulate food intake.

Osteoporosis: Calcium is essential for building and maintaining strong bones.

Ovarian cancer: Omega-3s, selenium, and other nutrients show benefits in slowing cell growth and boosting immunity.

Stroke: Eating two to four servings of fish a week reduces the risk of ischemic stroke by 18 percent.

HEALTH SPOTLIGHT

Omega-3s in Anchovies Reduce Cancer Tumor Size

Omega-3s are proving to be a promising ally in the fight against cancer. A 2009 study demonstrates that DHA, an omega-3 fatty acid found in anchovies and other fatty fish, can reduce tumor size in three ways: DHA was shown to attenuate tumor growth on a molecular level by reducing inflammation, slowing leukocytosis (the accumulation of white blood cells), and lessening oxidative stress.

QUICK TIPS

❖ Try this favorite Italian dip: This is an easy version of bagna càuda, which translates as *warm bath* in Italian. Simmer about ten finely chopped anchovies (one 2-ounce can) in $1/2$ cup olive oil for about 3 minutes. Add six cloves chopped garlic and simmer another 3 minutes or so until anchovies are dissolved. (Be careful not to burn the garlic.) Add $1/4$ cup unsalted butter (half a stick) and heat until melted. Try as a dip with cruciferous vegetables like broccoli and cauliflower, or with asparagus, artichokes, or toasted crostini.

❖ To give tomato-based pasta sauces more flavor, try adding a little anchovy paste (about $1/8$ teaspoon) or an equal amount of chopped anchovy.

Anchovy-Avocado Appetizer

YIELD: 8 SERVINGS

6 fresh plum tomatoes

1 2-ounce can anchovy fillets, packed in olive oil

2 garlic cloves, whole

$1/_4$ cup fresh squeezed lemon juice

Zest from squeezed lemons (zest before juicing)

2 cups mashed avocado

1 loaf multigrain flat bread or baguette

Olive oil

Preheat oven to 400°F. Position a cooling rack over a baking sheet. Remove the tomato stems and cut each tomato in half. Place the tomato halves cut-side down on the cooling rack. Place the baking sheet in the oven. Bake 20 to 30 minutes until the skins start to take on color and the flesh is soft. Allow them to cool, then remove and discard the skins. You should be able to pluck off the skins in one piece. Dice the tomatoes.

Place the garlic and the anchovies with their oil in the work bowl of a food processor. Process the mixture until minced. Add the lemon juice and zest. Process the mixture until you have a smooth sauce. Add the mashed avocado and pulse just until you have a smooth paste and all ingredients are well incorporated.

Cut the loaf of bread in half lengthwise. Brush the insides with olive oil. Heat a griddle over a medium-low flame. To toast the bread, place the bread, oiled sides down, on the warm griddle. Weigh the bread down with heavy cans. Toasting should take about 2 minutes.

Spread the avocado mixture on the toasted bread. Top the avocado with the roasted tomatoes. Cut the bread into eight slices and serve as an appetizer, light lunch, or first course.

＊　＊　＊

For more recipes using anchovies, see: Cucumber Relish (page 87), Tomato-Seafood Chowder (page 203).

4. APPLES

The famous expression "An apple a day keeps the doctor away" is said to have originated as a Welsh proverb in 1866: "Eat an apple on going to bed, and you'll keep the doctor from earning his bread." And although in the 1800s they may not have known the science behind exactly *why* apples kept one healthy, they must have seen the benefits. As far back as Hippocrates, who recommended them for digestive problems (he was right), apples have been associated with health. Today, research is uncovering the mysteries behind the amazing apple. Loaded with fiber, flavonoids, and vitamin C, apples are proving to fight an array of diseases including heart disease and Alzheimer's disease. Phytonutrients in apples, including quercetin, chlorogenic acid, phloridzin, and catechin, provide strong antioxidant protection—among the highest of any fruit.

HEALTH BENEFITS

Research shows compounds and nutrients found in apples may benefit:

Alzheimer's disease: Long-term consumption of fruit juice including apple juice proved to offer protection against this disease.

Asthma: Quercetin works to prevent immune cells from releasing histamines (chemicals that cause allergic reactions) and helps decrease symptoms like wheezing.

Breast cancer: Apple extract (equivalent to eating one to six apples daily) prevented breast cancer in animal studies; the more extract given, the greater the protection.

Cancer (colon and liver cancers): Apple extract was found to inhibit cancer cell proliferation in colon and liver cancers.

Cataracts associated with diabetes: Quercetin helps prevent cataracts from forming, possibly due to its cholesterol-lowering properties; high cholesterol levels are linked to cataracts.

Cholera: Apple extract has been shown to significantly inhibit the cholera toxin.

Digestive health: Insoluble apple fiber helps with constipation, beneficial in diverticulitis, while apple's pectin content can both help with constipation and, conversely, relieve diarrhea.

Eczema: Quercetin acts as an antihistamine and decreases symptoms like rash and itchy skin.

Hay fever: Quercetin helps prevent immune cells from releasing histamines that trigger allergic symptoms such as itchy, watery eyes and sneezing.

Heart disease: Quercetin and other flavonoids (found only in apple peel) lowered heart disease risk by up to 20 percent.

High cholesterol: Soluble and insoluble fiber work together to mop up LDL (bad) cholesterol and keep it from forming.

APPLES NUTRITION INFORMATION		
Serving Size 1 cup apple, quartered		
Amount Per Serving		
Calories 65	Calories from fat 2	
		% Daily Value*
Total Fat 0 grams		0%
Saturated fat 0 gm		0%
Trans fat 0 gm		†
Cholesterol 0 milligrams		0%
Sodium 1 mg		.04%
Total Carbohydrate 17 gm		6%
Dietary fiber 3 gm		12%
Sugars 13 gm		†
Protein 0 gm		0%
Vitamin A		1%
Vitamin C		10%
Calcium		1%
Iron		1%
Also contains:		
Potassium		4%
Phytosterols 15 mg		†
† Daily Value not established.		
* Percent Daily Values are based on a 2,000-calorie diet.		

Kidney stones: Drinking apple juice has been shown to increase urinary pH and citric acid excretion, decreasing chances of developing kidney stones.

Osteoporosis: Phloridzin (a flavonoid found only in apples) may prevent bone loss related to menopause and possibly increase bone density.

Prostate cancer: Quercetin may inhibit hormone activity in prostate cancer cell lines.

Type 2 diabetes: Apple fiber, plus the fructose (fruit sugar) in apples, breaks down slowly and does not spike blood sugar levels.

UVB protection: The Braeburn variety of apple protects its own skin from the sun by developing quercetin glycosides in its peel, which may in turn protect you from the burning ultraviolet B (UVB) spectrum of the sun's rays.

Viruses: Quercetin has antiviral properties that may prevent viruses, including herpes simplex and the flu, from reproducing inside cells.

Weight control: One study showed that people who ate an apple before meals consumed fewer calories.

HEALTH SPOTLIGHT

Artery Protection

A study of extracts from Fuji, Golden Delicious, Red Delicious, and Granny Smith apples showed that when added to endothelial cells (cells that make up the inner lining of arteries), they blocked chemical signals that lead to damage and inflammation in the arteries. The apple flavonoids prevented cells from damage by tumor necrosis factor (TNF), which induces a chemical signaling pathway that can lead to cell death, by inhibiting communications between the cells. This mechanism is known in addition to the antioxidant effects of the flavonoids in apples that prevent free radicals from damaging DNA.

QUICK TIP

❖ Pick Fuji or Red Delicious for the highest phytonutrient phenol and flavonoid content of popular apple varieties. Be sure to buy organic for higher antioxidant content and to avoid pesticide residues.

Roasted Pork Tenderloin with Apple-Brie Sauce and Apple-Almond Pilaf

YIELD: 4 SERVINGS

Pork Tenderloin
1 to 1$^1/_4$ pounds pork tenderloin

2 tablespoons grape seed oil

1 to 2 medium sweet onions (Maui or Vidalia),
weighing about 1 pound

Apple-Brie Sauce
3 Granny Smith apples, weighing about 1$^1/_2$ pounds,
peeled, cored, thinly sliced

1 teaspoon kosher salt

1 12-ounce bottle hard apple cider, at room temperature

1 cup evaporated milk

1 tablespoon Dijon mustard

$^1/_4$ teaspoon nutmeg

$^1/_4$ teaspoon black pepper

4 ounces Brie cheese, weighing 4 ounces after rind is removed

Salt and pepper to taste

Apple-Almond Pilaf
1 tablespoon grape seed oil

$^3/_4$ cup short-grain brown rice

$^1/_2$ cup minced dried apples

$^1/_4$ cup sliced almonds

2 cups hard apple cider

$^1/_2$ teaspoon salt

Preheat oven to 350°F. Pork tenderloin tends to have a tapered end. To ensure even cooking, fold the tapered end up so that the tenderloin has consistent thickness. Secure the end to the thicker portion with culinary twine. Season the tenderloin on all sides with a light sprinkling of salt and pepper. In a large skillet, over high heat, heat the grape seed oil and cook tenderloin to a golden brown on all sides.

Place the tenderloin on a rack positioned over a baking sheet. Insert a meat thermometer into the thickest portion of the tenderloin. Roast until the thermometer reads 160°F.

TO MAKE THE SAUCE: As the tenderloin roasts, in the same skillet in which you seared the tenderloin, cook the onions and apples with the 1 teaspoon kosher salt over a medium flame until they are soft and just starting to take on color. Add the cider to the pan. Cook until the cider is almost completely evaporated. There should be just a little bubbly moisture visible between the apples. At this point, remove from heat and wait to finish the sauce until the tenderloin has been removed from the oven.

When the internal temperature of the tenderloin is 160°F, remove it from the oven and let it rest, uncut, for 10 minutes. About 5 minutes before you are ready to serve the dish, heat the apple mixture over a low heat. Add the evaporated milk, mustard, nutmeg, black pepper, and Brie. Stir constantly over low heat just until the cheese has been completely incorporated. Salt and pepper to taste.

TO SERVE: Divide the apple mixture evenly among four plates. Remove the twine and slice the tenderloin. Divide the tenderloin slices among the four plates and fan the pieces of meat over the apple mixture. Serve with Apple-Almond Pilaf (directions below).

TO MAKE THE PILAF: Preheat oven to 350°F. In an ovenproof dish with a tight-fitting lid, combine the oil, rice, apples, and almonds. In a small saucepan, bring the cider and salt to a boil. Pour the cider over the rice mixture. Cover and bake for 70 minutes. Fluff with a fork and let it rest uncovered 5 minutes before serving.

* * *

For other recipes and ways of using apples, see: Mom's Red Cabbage (page 64), Carrot Griddle Cakes (page 68), Worth-the-Wait Caramelized Onion Bruschetta (page 146), Apple-Cinnamon Muesli (page 221).

5. APRICOTS

If the Hunza people of the Himalayas are any indication, apricots promote health and longevity. Legend has it that the Hunza (who eat apricots on a regular basis) remain healthy and vital into their nineties and beyond. Apricots are a member of the rose family, and have origins in China where they have been grown since 2,000 B.C. It is said that they were first brought to the West by Alexander the Great. They are rich in the carotenoids beta-cryptoxanthin as well as beta-carotene, a precursor for vitamin A. While fresh apricots are higher in vitamin C, dried apricots boast a higher calcium and iron content (the Hunza eat both). Both are a good source of fiber, which along with carotenoids and lycopene, account for much of the apricot's disease-fighting benefits. Best of all, they lend great flavor to sweet or savory dishes.

HEALTH BENEFITS

Research shows compounds and nutrients found in apricots may benefit:

Breast cancer: Lycopene shows promise in inhibiting breast cancer cell growth.

Cataracts: Vitamin A was found to reduce cataract risk by 39 percent.

Cognitive decline: Lycopene slows cognitive decline related to diabetes.

Colon cancer: Beta-cryptoxanthin shows benefit in fighting colon cancer, possibly by fending off free-radical damage to DNA; beta-carotene was found to reduce colon polyp risk in non-smokers by 40 percent.

Diverticulitis: Fiber helps promote healthy digestion, prevent constipation, and lower risk.

Fertility in men: Lycopene shows promise in promoting fertility in men.

Gallstones: Insoluble fiber speeds the transit time of food through the intestines while reducing bile acid secretion (which can lead to gallstones).

Gingivitis: Lycopene has antibacterial and antifungal properties that help prevent gum inflammation; vitamin C is also effective, especially for bleeding gums.

Heart disease: Fiber, beta-carotene, and lycopene help prevent heart disease by keeping LDL (bad) cholesterol from clogging arteries.

High blood pressure: Research shows both lycopene and potassium can lower blood pressure.

Kidney stones: Fiber may prevent crystallization of calcium, which can lead to stones; potassium may also inhibit crystallization and has been associated with a lower risk.

Lung cancer: Beta-cryptoxanthin shows benefit against lung cancer, possibly by shielding cells in sensitive lung tissue from free-radical damage.

Macular degeneration (age-related): Antioxidants and carotenoids work together to reduce free-radical damage; eating three or more servings of fruit a day may lower risk.

APRICOTS NUTRITION INFORMATION	
Serving Size $1/2$ cup apricots, dried	
Amount Per Serving	
Calories 156	Calories from fat 3
	% Daily Value*
Total Fat .5 grams	.5%
Saturated fat 0 gm	0%
Trans fat 0 gm	†
Cholesterol 0 milligrams	0%
Sodium 6.5 mg	.5%
Total Carbohydrate 40 gm	13.5%
Dietary fiber 4.5 gm	19%
Sugars 34.5 gm	†
Protein 2 gm	4%
Vitamin A	47%
Vitamin C	1%
Calcium	3.5%
Iron	9.5%
Also contains:	
Potassium	31%
† Daily Value not established.	
* Percent Daily Values are based on a 2,000-calorie diet.	

Night blindness: Beta-carotene may slow damage to the retina.

Prostate cancer: Regular consumption of lycopene-containing foods may lower prostate cancer risk by up to 82 percent!

Skin damage: Vitamin A offers some protection against harm from UV sunlight.

Type 2 diabetes: Fiber helps control blood sugar levels after meals by slowing the release of glucose into the bloodstream.

Weight loss and weight control: Fiber-containing foods provide a feeling of fullness; fiber slows digestion, helping to keep blood sugar levels stable and reduce insulin spikes that can trigger cravings and encourage fat storage.

HEALTH SPOTLIGHT

Reduce Risk of Cataracts

A study that monitored the diets of 50,000 women showed a correlation between high vitamin A intake and reduced risk of developing cataracts. In fact, women who consumed the most vitamin A from foods including apricots reduced their risk by almost 40 percent.

QUICK TIP

❖ To prolong the shelf life of dried apricots, refrigerate them. They can be stored for about six months in the refrigerator versus one month at room temperature and will retain more nutrients.

Apricot Moroccan-Style Stew

YIELD: 8 SERVINGS

2 pounds stewing beef or lamb steak cut into cubes

2 to 4 tablespoons olive oil

1 pound sweet onions (Maui or Vidalia), thinly sliced

3 to 4 large cloves of garlic, crushed

8 ounces baby carrots

2 cups cabernet sauvignon wine

56 ounces canned, diced tomatoes

8 ounces dried apricots

$3/4$ teaspoon ground ginger

$1/2$ teaspoon allspice

$1 1/2$ teaspoons cinnamon

$1/2$ teaspoon nutmeg

1 teaspoon smoked paprika

2 tablespoons honey

Salt and pepper

Whole-wheat couscous

Preheat oven to 325°F. In a 5-quart Dutch oven, over a high flame, heat about 2 tablespoons of olive oil. Season the meat liberally with salt and pepper. In batches, being careful not to crowd the pan, brown the meat. Place browned meat on a plate and wrap it with foil. Once all the meat has been browned, reduce the heat in the pan to low. Add the onions, garlic, and carrots to the pot. Add more oil if necessary. Cook, stirring every few minutes, until the onions are soft and have begun to take on some color. When you stir, scrape the bottom of the pot to loosen and incorporate the residue left by the meat. Add the wine and return the flame to high. Bring to a vigorous boil. Stir in the tomatoes, apricots, ginger, allspice, cinnamon, nutmeg, paprika, honey, and the browned meat. Once again bring to a vigorous boil.

Cover and place in the oven. Braise the stew in the oven for 2 hours. When ready to serve, prepare whole-wheat couscous according to the package directions. Ladle the stew over the couscous in a soup bowl.

6. ARUGULA

Arugula was considered an aphrodisiac by the ancient Egyptians and Romans who associated it with a Roman god of fertility. Perhaps it is the folate and manganese in arugula, both nutrients linked to sexual health, which helped to earn it this reputation. This leafy vegetable entices the senses with its peppery taste and aroma, spicing up salads, pastas, soups, and more, and is especially popular in Italy where it is considered a very common garden green. Like other members of the cruciferous vegetable family, arugula is high in glucosinolates that act as powerful cancer fighters. And arugula is an excellent source of vitamin K, in addition to containing beta-carotene, calcium, lutein, zeaxanthin, and phytochemicals such as chlorophyll, quercetin, and kaempferol. All for just 2 calories per half cup!

HEALTH BENEFITS

Research shows compounds and nutrients found in arugula may benefit:

Asthma: Quercetin works to prevent immune cells from releasing histamines (chemicals that cause allergic reactions) and may decrease symptoms like wheezing.

Bladder cancer: Eating a diet that includes plenty of cruciferous vegetables may cut the risk of bladder cancer by 29 percent.

Cancer (breast, colon, lung, prostate, and stomach cancers, and non-Hodgkin's lymphoma): Cruciferous vegetables have been shown to protect cells from oxidants associated with these cancers (see Health Spotlight); glucosinolates and chlorophyll aid in the detoxification of carcinogens that can lead to cancer.

Cataracts: Vitamin A and beta-carotene are associated with reduced risk of vision-clouding cataracts.

Depression: Kaempferol acts as an antidepressant.

Eczema: Quercetin acts as an anti-histamine and may decrease symptoms like rash and itchy skin.

Fatigue: Iron combats anemia that can lead to fatigue and low energy.

Flu: Quercetin is associated with increased protection against the flu virus.

Hay fever: Quercetin helps prevent immune cells from releasing histamines that trigger allergic symptoms such as itchy, watery eyes and sneezing.

Macular degeneration (age-related): Lutein, zeaxanthin, and carotenoids help retain macular pigments in the eye, and antioxidants reduce free-radical damage.

Osteoporosis: Calcium, manganese, and vitamin K work synergistically to build bone and protect it from weakening or fracturing.

Ovarian cancer: Kaempferol is associated with a 40 percent lower risk of ovarian cancer; evidence suggests the flavonoid's antioxidant activity may inhibit the development of cancer cells.

Prostate cancer: Quercetin may inhibit hormone activity in prostate cancer cell lines.

Varicose veins: Vitamin K promotes healthy blood clotting and is associated with fewer varicose veins; rutin contributes by strengthening capillaries.

ARUGULA NUTRITION INFORMATION

Serving Size 1/2 cup arugula (10 g)

Amount Per Serving

Calories 2 — Calories from fat 0

	% Daily Value*
Total Fat 0 grams	0%
Saturated fat 0 gm	0%
Trans fat 0 gm	†
Cholesterol 0 milligrams	0%
Sodium 3 mg	.125%
Total Carbohydrate 0 gm	0%
Dietary fiber 0 gm	0%
Sugars 0 gm	†
Protein 0 gm	0%
Vitamin A	5%
Vitamin C	2%
Calcium	2%
Iron	1%
Also contains:	
Vitamin K	14%
Folate	2%
Manganese	2%

† Daily Value not established.
* Percent Daily Values are based on a 2,000-calorie diet.

HEALTH SPOTLIGHT

Potent Cancer Fighter

In the Nurses' Health Study, those who consumed the highest amounts of cruciferous vegetables such as arugula (five or more servings a week) showed a 33 percent lower risk of developing non-Hodgkin's lymphoma (a cancer that starts in the lymph system).

QUICK TIPS

❖ Use arugula in place of lettuce on sandwiches.

❖ Mix chopped arugula in mayo.

❖ Try arugula as an alternative to basil in pesto sauce.

Arugula Brunch Stack

YIELD: 4 SERVINGS

3 tablespoons safflower or canola mayonnaise

1 tablespoon Dijon mustard

1 tablespoon finely minced shallot

1 tablespoon lemon juice

1 cup baby arugula

4 slices Canadian bacon

4 slices (about 1-inch thick) whole multigrain
artesian loaf bread

4 slices (about $1/4$-inch thick) from a large
heirloom tomato

4 slices (about $1/2$ ounce each) cheddar cheese

4 eggs

Nonstick cooking spray

In a large bowl combine the mayonnaise, mustard, shallot, and lemon juice. Toss the arugula in the dressing to coat well. Set aside.

Toast the slices of bread. Meanwhile, warm the Canadian bacon in a skillet.

To assemble, put one slice of bread on each plate. Top the bread with one-quarter of the dressed arugula, then one slice of tomato and one slice of cheese. Place the warm Canadian bacon on top of the cheese. In a skillet prepared with nonstick cooking spray, cook each egg either sunny-side up or over-easy. Top the stack with one hot egg and serve immediately.

* * *

For other recipes and ways of using arugula, see: Quinoa-Chicken Salad (page 169), Tuna Tartare Appetizer Salad (page 208).

7. ASPARAGUS

"Asparagus inspires gentle thoughts."
—Charles Lamb, English poet (1775–1834)

With origins in the Mediterranean dating back thousands of years, asparagus is a true "Mediterranean diet" vegetable. It is thought to have been cultivated by the ancient Egyptians, and was harvested by the ancient Romans, who ate it fresh and even dried it so they could enjoy it out of season. It had medicinal purposes for the Greeks, who used it for stomach and bowel ailments, as a diuretic, and to remove obstructions from the liver and kidneys. Anecdotal reports even suggest it can cure cancer! (And research supports asparagus as a cancer fighter.) Loaded with vitamin K, the minerals folate and iron, as well as compounds like arginine and asparagine (both amino acids), glutathione (a phytochemical that acts as an antioxidant), rutin (a flavonoid), and methylsulfonylmethane (or MSM, a sulfur compound), asparagus is proving to have many of the attributes that have long been believed.

HEALTH BENEFITS

Research shows compounds and nutrients found in asparagus may benefit:

Allergies: MSM reduces inflammation, possibly by reducing toxins in cells.

Cancer (lung, breast, and bladder cancers): Glutathione has shown preventive effects against these cancers.

Cognitive function: Arginine converts to nitric oxide to relax blood vessels and improve blood flow to the brain; iron is linked to enhanced brain function.

Depression: Low levels of B-complex vitamins are linked to depression; B vitamins are necessary for the synthesis of the feel-good chemical serotonin that helps regulate anxiety and mood.

Detox: Asparagine's diuretic effects aid in detoxification.

Edema, or swelling from fluid retention: Asparagine acts as a diuretic, helping to flush excess water from the body; rutin may reduce swelling.

Erectile dysfunction: Arginine changes to nitric oxide, which causes blood-vessel relaxation and increases blood flow.

Flu: Rutin acts as an antiviral; in studies, flavonoids like rutin have demonstrated antiviral activity on herpes simplex and even HIV.

Heart health: Folate helps metabolize homocysteine (an amino acid that increases heart-disease risk when levels build up in the blood); glutathione protects against the formation of arterial plaque; arginine, which converts to nitric oxide, relaxes blood vessels and increases blood flow.

Hemorrhoids: Rutin helps to strengthen the capillaries around hemorrhoids and keeps tissue from breaking down.

High blood pressure: Potassium lowers blood pressure.

High cholesterol: Sterols and saponins work to lower cholesterol by blocking its absorption in the intestines, while polyphenols, flavonoids, and vitamin C may inhibit oxidation of harmful LDL cholesterol and plaque buildup.

ASPARAGUS NUTRITION INFORMATION

Serving Size 1 cup asparagus, uncooked

Amount Per Serving

Calories 27	Calories from fat 1
	% Daily Value*
Total Fat 0 grams	0%
Saturated fat 0 gm	0%
Trans fat 0 gm	†
Cholesterol 0 milligrams	0%
Sodium 3 mg	.125%
Total Carbohydrate 5 gm	2%
Dietary fiber 3 gm	11%
Sugars 3 gm	†
Protein 3 gm	6%
Vitamin A	20%
Vitamin C	13%
Calcium	3%
Iron	16%
Also contains:	
Vitamin K	70%
Folate	17%
Vitamin B$_1$ (thiamine)	13%
Copper	13%
Vitamin B$_2$ (riboflavin)	11%
Manganese	11%
Potassium	8%
Vitamin E	8%

† Daily Value not established.
* Percent Daily Values are based on a 2,000-calorie diet.

Immunity: Rutin and vitamin C boost immune function.

Irritable bowel syndrome: Inulin increases healthy bacteria in the intestines that may help lessen IBS-related gas, pain, and bloating (see Health Spotlight).

Kidney stones: An association between vitamin E and reduced risk factors for kidney stones was found in one study, although the mechanism is not known.

Libido: Folate boosts histamine, necessary for sexual function, and vitamin E enhances libido, possibly by encouraging healthy circulation.

Liver health: Glutathione and folic acid may reduce liver damage from cancer medications.

Macular degeneration (age-related): Studies show B vitamins can lower risk; glutathione protects the tissues of the eye lens and is associated with improved vision.

Osteo- and rheumatoid arthritis: MSM decreases inflammation and may be effective in reducing pain and increasing joint function.

Osteoporosis: Vitamin K helps improve bone density, in part, by slowing calcium loss in bone.

Pregnancy: Folate serves a critical function in growth and reproduction, and protects against a number of congenital malformations, including neural tube birth defects.

PMS symptoms: Asparagine acts as a diuretic to help reduce premenstrual bloating.

Stroke: Glutathione's antioxidant activity may assist in recovery from stroke.

Ulcers: Glutathione guards against infection from *H. pylori* bacteria that cause peptic ulcers.

Varicose veins: Vitamin K promotes healthy blood clotting and is associated with fewer varicose veins; rutin contributes by strengthening capillaries.

HEALTH SPOTLIGHT

Asparagus Benefits IBS

It seems the Greeks were right about asparagus' powers to provide relief for stomach and bowel problems. Asparagus contains inulin, a prebiotic carbohydrate that we don't digest, but the friendly bacteria in our intestines thrive on. Prebiotics have shown promise in benefiting irritable bowel syndrome (IBS). "Good" bacteria such as bifidobacteria and lactobacilli in our large intestine increase when more inulin is consumed in the diet, making survival more difficult for the unfriendly bacteria in the gut that can cause digestive problems.

QUICK TIPS

❖ It is said that one of Roman emperor Augustus' favorite expressions was, "Quicker than you can cook asparagus!" Before cooking, chop off the ends of the stalks, or break them off by hand (the stalks will naturally bend at the right spot).

❖ For asparagus "fries," roast asparagus in a shallow pan with a little olive oil, salt, and pepper in a 350°F oven until the tips are slightly browned and crispy. This gives asparagus a slightly nutty flavor. (Try this with the anchovy dip on page 14.)

❖ Chop leftover asparagus into pasta or omelets.

Creamy Asparagus Soup

YIELD: 6 SERVINGS

6 tablespoons olive oil

1 large brown onion, thinly sliced

5 large cloves garlic, peeled and crushed

1 pound asparagus, roughly chopped but not peeled

2 tablespoons soy sauce

1 cup chardonnay or other dry white wine

6 cups homemade or canned low-sodium chicken broth

1 cup instant mashed potato flakes

12 ounces evaporated milk

Heat the oil, on low, in a large skillet. Add the onions, garlic, and asparagus. Cook the vegetables, stirring every few minutes until they are very soft and are just starting to take on color, about 20 minutes. Add the soy sauce and chardonnay. Continue to cook over low heat, stirring occasionally, until the liquid has been reduced by about three-fourths its original volume.

Transfer the vegetable/wine mixture to the jar of a blender in batches. Blend until liquefied. You may need to add some of the chicken broth to make the vegetables loose enough to be liquefied. Force the liquefied vegetables through a fine mesh sieve. Discard any fibrous mass that will not go through the sieve. Repeat this process until all the vegetables have been liquefied and run through the sieve.

Transfer soup to a stockpot with any remaining broth. Bring it back up to a simmer and add the potato flakes. Whisk until flakes have been completely incorporated. Stir in evaporated milk. Heat and serve.

*   *   *

For other ways of using asparagus, see: Anchovy Quick Tips (page 14).

8. AVOCADOS

The avocado originated in Mexico where the Aztecs associated it with fertility. In fact, the Aztec word for avocado was *ahuacatl,* which translates as "testicle." (Since then, it has been discovered that the avocado does contain nutrients known to benefit reproductive health as well as boost libido.) After the Spanish invasion, ahuacatl became *aguacate,* and eventually avocado in English. Avocados have been a part of Mexican cooking for centuries, dating as far back as 500 B.C., but have found their way into Asian, Italian, and even Indian fare. From garnishing soups to topping burgers, the beloved avocado is incredibly versatile in addition to being a nutritional powerhouse. A single avocado packs a wallop of vitamins and minerals, antioxidants including glutathione, carotenoids such as lutein and zeaxanthin, and fiber. And nevermind the fat content—healthy fats including oleic acid (an omega-9 fatty acid) are known to benefit the heart and help you absorb nutrients.

HEALTH BENEFITS

Research shows compounds and nutrients found in avocados may benefit:

Aging and skin health: Vitamins C and E fight cellular aging by defending cell membranes against free-radical damage.

Alzheimer's disease: Eating a diet high in folate was found to lower Alzheimer's risk by half.

Anxiety: Omega-3s may be effective in reducing anxiety.

Attention deficit/hyperactivity disorder: Omega-3 fatty acids are linked with reduced symptoms and are often deficient in those with ADHD.

Breast cancer: Research shows omega-9s kill breast cancer cells.

Colorectal cancer: Vitamin B_6 was found to lower colorectal cancer risk, especially in women who drink alcohol, possibly by prohibiting cell proliferation and oxidative stress.

Depression: Omega-3s may be effective in lifting depression and boosting mood.

Digestive health: Fiber improves digestion and is linked to a reduced risk of hemorrhoids and diverticulitis (bulging tissue pouches in the colon).

Eye health: Lutein and zeaxanthin, which are concentrated in the macula, help enhance eyesight and protect against free radical damage caused by exposure to sunlight.

Healthy hair and skin color: Copper helps to produce melanin, the pigment responsible for hair and skin color.

Heart attack: Folate, which lowered heart attack risk by 55 percent in one study, inhibits the formation of homocysteine (a potentially toxic chemical and significant risk factor for heart disease).

Heart health: Research shows omega-3s help to improve triglyceride levels, stabilize heartbeat, lower blood pressure, and inhibit inflammation.

High blood pressure: Potassium lowers blood pressure.

AVOCADOS NUTRITION INFORMATION	
Serving Size 1 medium avocado	
Amount Per Serving	
Calories 322	Calories from fat 247
	% Daily Value*
Total Fat 29 grams	45%
Saturated fat gm	21%
Trans fat 0 gm	†
Cholesterol 0 milligrams	0%
Sodium 14 mg	1%
Total Carbohydrate 17 gm	6%
Dietary fiber 13 gm	54%
Sugars 1 gm	†
Protein 4 gm	8%
Vitamin A	4%
Vitamin C	33%
Calcium	2%
Iron	6%
Also contains:	
Vitamin K	53%
Folate	41%
Vitamin B_5 (pantothenic acid)	28%
Potassium	28%
Vitamin B_6 (pyridoxine)	26%
Vitamin E	21%
Copper	19%
Magnesium	15%
Omega-3 fatty acids 221 mg	†
Omega-6 fatty acids 3,396 mg	†
† Daily Value not established.	
* Percent Daily Values are based on a 2,000-calorie diet.	

Libido: Vitamin C is essential for the formation of androgen, estrogen, and progesterone—hormones related to libido; vitamin E is essential for the formation of hormone-like substances called prostaglandins that play a key role in desire; and B vitamins are essential for nerve health and energy.

Oral cancer: Phytonutrients including lutein target free radicals, possibly attenuating cell damage that can contribute to cancer.

Osteoporosis: Potassium and magnesium are necessary for maintaining strong bones; vitamin K helps by mobilizing calcium into bones.

Pancreatic cancer: One study showed a 59 percent decreased risk in people who ate foods high in folate, and an 81 percent decreased risk in those who ate foods high in vitamin B_6.

PMS symptoms: Magnesium helps alleviate irritability, bloating, and cramps associated with premenstrual syndrome.

Pregnancy: Folate serves a critical function in growth and reproduction, and protects against a number of congenital malformations, including neural tube birth defects.

Prostate cancer: A mix of lutein and other carotenoids, vitamin E, and healthy dietary fats, act together to protect against prostate cancer (see Health Spotlight).

Skin aging: Omega-6 fatty acids help maintain the skin's natural oil barrier, keeping skin soft and supple.

Stroke: Potassium lowers blood pressure and reduces the stickiness of blood platelets that can cause clots.

Wound healing: Pantothenic acid accelerates healing of skin injuries, including burns.

HEALTH SPOTLIGHT

Protection Against Prostate Cancer

Avocados contain lutein, other carotenoids including zeaxanthin and beta-carotene, the tocopherol vitamin E, plus healthy dietary fats that work together to protect against prostate cancer. In a study published in the *Journal of Nutri-*

tional Biochemistry, this combination of nutrients stopped the growth of prostate cancer cells. However, when lutein alone was tested, it had no effect on cancer cells. It is likely that rather than the nutrients in avocados working in isolation, it is the whole matrix of tocopherols and carotenoids plus the fat found in avocados (which ensures absorption of fat-soluble carotenoids into the bloodstream) that work as a cancer-fighting team.

QUICK TIPS

❖ Use mashed avocado in place of mayonnaise on sandwiches or wraps.

❖ Add diced avocado to fruit salads (avocados complement papaya, mango, and citrus fruits).

❖ Enhance carotenoid absorption from foods like spinach and tomatoes by adding avocado to salads and salsa.

❖ In baked goods such as muffins, mashed avocado may be substituted for half the butter called for.

Avocado-Tuna Wraps

YIELD: 4 SANDWICH WRAPS

Dressing
2 tablespoons safflower or canola mayonnaise

2 tablespoons fresh squeezed lime juice

Zest from squeezed lime (zest before juicing)

1 tablespoon minced cilantro

1 tablespoon (or to taste) minced chipotle in adobo sauce

Salad
1 7.5-ounce can of tuna, drained and flaked

$1/2$ cup cherub tomatoes, quartered, or about 6 cherry tomatoes diced small

3 scallions, green and white parts, thinly sliced

4 leaves red leaf lettuce

1 large avocado, sliced

4 7-inch multigrain tortillas

TO MAKE THE DRESSING: In a medium bowl, whisk the mayonnaise, lime juice, zest, cilantro, and chipotle.

TO MAKE THE SALAD: Add the tuna, tomatoes, and scallions, and toss well.

TO MAKE THE WRAPS: Lay one lettuce leaf in the center of each tortilla. On top of the lettuce, fan $1/4$ of the avocado slices. On top of the avocado, spread $1/4$ of the tuna salad. Roll the tortilla to encase the filling. Secure with a toothpick.

*   *   *

For other recipes and ways of using avocado, see: Anchovy-Avocado Appetizer (page 15), Black Bean Burritos with Spicy Chili Salsa (page 77), Tuna Tartare Appetizer Salad (page 208).

9. BANANAS

"Yeah, I like cars and basketball.
But you know what I like more? Bananas."
—FRANKIE MUNIZ, ACTOR

Bananas are well known for being high in potassium, but that's not the whole story. There are a bunch of benefits to be had from eating bananas. While a medium-sized banana does contain 12 percent of your daily requirement for potassium, it is even higher in vitamin C (17 percent), and it contains 22 percent vitamin B_6 (pyridoxine), and a range of other important B vitamins. Not only that, but bananas are loaded with flavonoids, fructooligosaccharides (FOS), and fiber, too. The vitamin B_6 in bananas may assist in controlling dandruff and fighting insomnia. And anecdotal reports claim this fruit is the perfect hangover cure. (In fact, there are nutrients in bananas that work to fight headaches and may reduce nausea.) Studies reveal even more amazing ways bananas keep us healthy.

HEALTH BENEFITS

Research shows compounds and nutrients found in bananas may benefit:

Attention deficit/hyperactivity disorder: Vitamin B_6, which is important for brain function, and magnesium, which has a calming effect, were found to decrease hyperactivity.

Bone health: FOS helps the body absorb calcium (see Health Spotlight).

Cancer: Beta-carotene and vitamin A may prevent free-radical damage to cell membranes and DNA.

Colon cancer: Research shows FOS and probiotics work synergistically to reduce tumors and lesions and slow cancer growth.

Depression: B vitamins assist the brain in producing mood-improving brain chemicals.

Diarrhea: Potassium helps replace lost electrolytes, fiber helps absorb liquid in the intestines, and FOS helps promote the growth of beneficial bacteria (probiotics) in the intestinal tract and balance gut flora.

Digestive health: Bananas contain a soluble fiber called hydrocolloid that has prebiotic effects.

Energy: B vitamins boost energy, while natural sugars plus fiber supply sustained energy.

Heart health: Potassium lowers blood pressure; fiber mops up artery-clogging cholesterol and shuttles it out of the body.

Kidney health: Regular consumption of bananas was found to reduce kidney cancer risk, possibly due to phenolic compounds that act as antioxidants.

Leg cramps: Potassium may alleviate leg cramps associated with pregnancy.

BANANAS NUTRITION INFORMATION	
Serving Size 1 medium banana	
Amount Per Serving	
Calories 105	Calories from fat 3
	% Daily Value*
Total Fat 0 grams	0%
Saturated fat 0 gm	0%
Trans fat 0 gm	†
Cholesterol 0 milligrams	0%
Sodium 1 mg	.04%
Total Carbohydrate 27 gm	9%
Dietary fiber 3 gm	12%
Sugars 14 gm	†
Protein 1 gm	2%
Vitamin A	2%
Vitamin C	17%
Calcium	1%
Iron	2%
Also contains:	
Vitamin B$_6$ (pyridoxine)	22%
Manganese	16%
Potassium	12%
Magnesium	8%
† Daily Value not established.	
* Percent Daily Values are based on a 2,000-calorie diet.	

Macular degeneration (age-related): Vitamins A and C protect the eyes from free-radical damage caused by exposure to sunlight.

Migraine headache: Magnesium relaxes muscles and nerves and is often low in migraine sufferers.

PMS symptoms: Symptoms are more common in women with low levels of magnesium, which helps to keep muscles from cramping.

Skin health: Vitamin C aids in collagen formation and protects against free-radical damage.

Stroke: Potassium and magnesium promote normal blood pressure and are associated with lower risk of stroke.

Type 2 diabetes: Carotenoids have been shown to have a positive effect on insulin resistance.

Ulcers: Protease inhibitors in bananas kill *H. pylori* bacteria in the stomach that cause peptic ulcers.

HEALTH SPOTLIGHT

Better Bone Health with Bananas

Here's a good reason to add sliced bananas to your breakfast cereal: Bananas help the body absorb nutrients including calcium, according to a study published in *Digestive Diseases and Sciences*. Bananas are an excellent source of FOS, a prebiotic that nourishes friendly bacteria in the gut. These beneficial bacteria produce vitamins and digestive enzymes that improve the ability to absorb nutrients like calcium, directly linked to better bone health. Green bananas also contain short-chain fatty acids that feed the cells in the lining of the intestines making them better able to absorb nutrients.

QUICK TIP

❖ Elvis was on to something with his famous fried banana and peanut butter sandwich. For a super-energy boost, make a healthier version of the Elvis sandwich with all-natural peanut butter, mashed or sliced bananas, and whole-wheat bread toasted instead of fried. Add honey or agave if desired.

Banana Upside-Down Breakfast Cake

YIELD: 8 SERVINGS

2 cups whole-wheat flour

1 teaspoon baking powder

$1/_2$ teaspoon salt

$1 1/_2$ teaspoons cardamom

1 teaspoon nutmeg

$^1/_2$ teaspoon allspice

$^1/_4$ teaspoon ground chipotle pepper

$^1/_2$ cup safflower oil

$1^1/_4$ cups agave nectar

2 teaspoons vanilla extract

2 eggs, beaten

$1^1/_2$ cups mashed very ripe bananas

$^3/_4$ cup whipping cream

Pinch salt

3 medium-sized very ripe bananas,
thinly sliced (about 12 ounces)

Preheat oven to 350°F. In a large bowl, combine the flour, baking powder, salt, cardamom, nutmeg, allspice, and chipotle pepper. Set aside.

In a medium-sized bowl, combine the oil, $^3/_4$ cup agave nectar, vanilla, eggs, and bananas. Set aside.

Spray an 8-by-8-inch baking pan with nonstick cooking spray.

In a medium skillet, combine the remaining agave nectar ($^1/_2$ cup), cream, and salt. Bring to a boil. Simmer, stirring frequently, over medium heat just until it starts to take on a caramel color and thicken slightly, about 7 minutes. Pour the hot caramel into the prepared baking pan. Fan the sliced bananas in the caramel to create a pattern.

Dump the oil/egg/banana mixture into the flour and spice mixture. Stir just enough to wet all the dry ingredients. Gently spoon the batter over the bananas and caramel, being careful not to disturb the pattern you created. Bake on the top rack of the oven with a large baking sheet underneath it to catch any drips. Bake for 45 to 55 minutes, until a toothpick inserted into the center of the cake comes out clean.

Cool on a wire cooling rack for 10 minutes. Place a large platter over the cake and invert it. Remove the pan. Spoon any runny sauce back over the top of the cake.

* * *

For other recipes and ways of using banana, see: Millet Quick Tips (page 128).

10. BEETS

For many of us, our first taste of beets was probably the canned variety, which doesn't really do the beet justice when it comes to bringing out the natural flavor. For this reason, we may have grown up wrinkling our noses at beets. But perhaps we should take a cue from the Russians. In a country famous for its borscht (beet soup), and where pickled beets are a dietary staple, living to 100 is not uncommon. Perhaps beets have something to do with the many Russian centenarians. Who knows? But we do know the beet is one of the healthiest vegetables around. Researchers have discovered several ways the compounds in beets work to protect the body. For example, betacyanin, the pigment in the beet that gives it its purple color, has proven to be a powerful cancer fighter. A metabolite in beets called betaine works to combat inflammation in the body. Add to that fiber and a healthy dose of vitamins and minerals, and the beet is worth a second look.

HEALTH BENEFITS

Research shows compounds and nutrients found in beets may benefit:

Alzheimer's disease: Betaine may prevent the formation of amyloid beta plaque that results in brain-cell damage.

Colon cancer: Betacyanin was found to inhibit cell mutations in the colon.

Common cold: Vitamin C boosts the immune system to fend off colds and reduce the duration of colds.

Gingivitis: Vitamin C promotes healing, especially of bleeding gums.

Heart disease: People whose diets contained plenty of betaine- and choline-rich foods showed lower levels of C-reactive protein, homocysteine, and other markers indicating inflammation than those whose diets did not.

High blood pressure: Potassium lowers blood pressure.

Osteo- and rheumatoid arthritis: Betaine inhibits inflammation (see Heart Disease).

Osteoporosis: Manganese is important for bone growth.

Pregnancy: Folate serves a critical function in growth and reproduction, and protects against a number of congenital malformations, including neural tube birth defects.

PMS symptoms: Manganese, taken with calcium, may reduce cramps.

Psoriasis: Betaine inhibits inflammation (see Heart Disease).

Stomach cancer: Betacyanin inhibits cancer-causing nitrosamines from forming.

Stroke: Potassium lowers blood pressure and reduces the stickiness of blood platelets that can cause clots.

Type 2 diabetes: Fiber helps control blood sugar levels after meals by slowing the release of glucose into the bloodstream.

Weight loss and weight control: Fiber-containing foods provide a feeling of fullness; fiber slows digestion, helping to keep blood sugar levels stable and reduce insulin spikes that can trigger cravings and encourage fat storage.

BEETS NUTRITION INFORMATION

Serving Size 1 beet, raw

Amount Per Serving

Calories 35	Calories from fat 1
	% Daily Value*
Total Fat 0 grams	0%
Saturated fat 0 gm	0%
Trans fat 0 gm	†
Cholesterol 0 milligrams	0%
Sodium 64 mg	3%
Total Carbohydrate 8 gm	3%
Dietary fiber 2 gm	9%
Sugars 6 gm	†
Protein 1 gm	2%
Vitamin A	1%
Vitamin C	7%
Calcium	1%
Iron	4%
Also contains:	
Folate	22%
Manganese	13%
Potassium	8%

† Daily Value not established.
* Percent Daily Values are based on a 2,000-calorie diet.

HEALTH SPOTLIGHT

Beets Guard Against Inflammatory Diseases

Chronic inflammation in the body, which can be triggered by causes such as stress, poor diet, or infection, is associated with numerous diseases. Inflammation can lead to heart disease, osteo- and rheumatoid arthritis, and Alzheimer's disease, just to name a few. However, a compound in beets offers a way to fight back. A study published in the *American Journal of Clinical Nutrition* found that people whose diets supplied the highest average intake of betaine (a metabolite found in beets) showed significantly lower signs of inflammation— at least 20 percent lower—than those with the lowest average intake.

QUICK TIPS

❖ Juice raw beets for a super-nutrition boost.

❖ Grate raw beets and toss them into salads.

❖ Don't throw away the green leafy tops—they can be eaten, too! Discard the stems, wash and chop the leaves, and sauté them in olive oil and garlic for a quick side dish. Add salt and pepper to taste.

Roasted Beet and Fennel Salad

YIELD: 4 APPETIZER SALADS

Beets

1 bunch or 3 large beets (about 1 pound)

Greens from beets, cut into a chiffonade (see directions on page 46)

$1/4$ cup olive oil

2 teaspoons kosher salt

Dressing

3 tablespoons thawed orange juice concentrate

3 tablespoons olive oil

3 tablespoons apple cider vinegar

$1/2$ teaspoon kosher salt

Zest from two oranges

Salad

1 fennel bulb, fronds and core removed, thinly sliced

2 large oranges, supremed (see directions on page 47)

Preheat oven to 350°F.

TO PREPARE THE BEETS: Peel the beets and remove the tops and bottoms. Wash and reserve the beet greens for later use. Dice the beets into large $1/2$-inch cubes. In a large mixing bowl, combine $1/4$ cup of olive oil and 2 teaspoons of salt. Toss this mixture with the beets to coat. Line a baking sheet with a sheet of aluminum foil. Spread the beets evenly over the foil leaving a 1-inch border unused. Top the beets with another piece of foil. Crimp the edges of the two sheets of foil to create an envelope for the beets. Bake them for 1 hour.

TO MAKE THE DRESSING: In a small bowl, combine the orange juice concentrate, 3 tablespoons of olive oil, vinegar, $1/2$ teaspoon of salt, and orange zest. Whisk well and set aside.

While the beets are still hot transfer them to a heat-safe bowl. Pour the dressing over the beets and toss together to marinate. Chill in the refrigerator until cool, or overnight.

TO MAKE THE SALAD: Make a chiffonade of the beet greens and supreme the oranges.

A Chiffonade of Leafy Greens

To make a chiffonade of leafy greens, wash and dry the greens. Stack the leaves one on top of another, and roll them tightly. Using a sharp knife, slice the leaves across the roll to create long thin pieces.

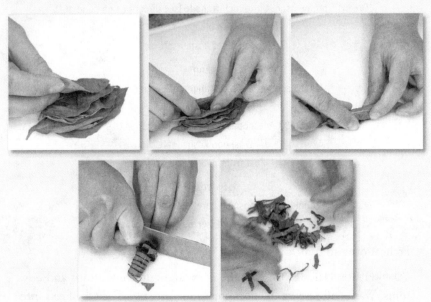

Place the greens on a large serving platter. Top with the sliced fennel, then the orange supremes. Arrange the marinated beets on top of the greens with the fennel and oranges, and dress with the remaining marinade.

To Supreme Citrus Fruit

A supreme is a segment of orange (or any other citrus fruit) without pith, skin, or membrane. Cut off just enough of the top and bottom of the orange so that the flesh is visible and the pith is removed. Set the fruit on one of the flat sides you have created. Follow the curvature of the fruit with the blade of your knife and remove a section of the pith and peel, leaving the flesh intact. Rotate the fruit after each slice and repeat until you have removed all of the peel. Using the membrane as a guide, cut out each section of the orange. Use two small cuts to create a v-shape. Discard the empty membranes.

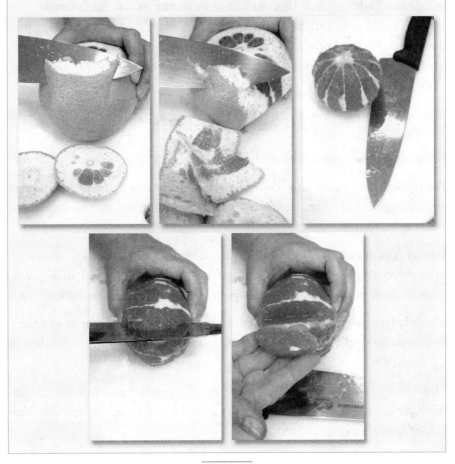

11. BLACK BEANS

Excavations of prehistoric dwellings in Central and South America have found evidence that black beans were a staple food as far back as 7,000 years ago. From the Americas where they originated, they have become popular throughout the world, especially in Latin American, Caribbean, and Asian cooking. Black beans are a super-energy food, loaded with protein, "good" carbs and fiber, and low in fat. When combined with a whole grain such as brown rice, the protein profile is comparable to meat. Black beans also contain compounds called anthocyanins and polyphenols that act as antioxidants—in fact, they have as much antioxidant power as grapes and cranberries. Their dark color indicates a higher antioxidant content than lighter beans. Additionally, they are high in the trace mineral manganese, which plays a key role in energy production and acts as a cofactor in the production of a scavenger enzyme called superoxide dismutase (SOD) that neutralizes harmful free radicals.

HEALTH BENEFITS

Research shows compounds and nutrients found in black beans may benefit:

Brain health: Protein and B-complex vitamins, especially folate, protect against cognitive decline; iron is associated with improved concentration and memory in women.

Cancer (colon and liver cancers): A phytochemical in beans called diosgenin may prevent cancer cells from multiplying; anthocyanins and other compounds work synergistically to offer protection (see Health Spotlight).

Chronic fatigue syndrome: Magnesium is needed for the synthesis of adenosine triphosphate (ATP, a primary energy source for cells), and is often low in CFS sufferers.

Depression: Low levels of B-complex vitamins are linked to depression; B vitamins are necessary for the synthesis of the feel-good chemical serotonin that helps regulate anxiety and mood.

Diverticulitis: Fiber helps promote healthy digestion, prevent constipation, and lower risk.

Energy: Iron helps red blood cells carry oxygen to cells and protects against anemia associated with low energy.

Gallstones: Insoluble fiber speeds the transit of food through the intestines while reducing bile acid secretion (which can lead to gallstones).

Heart attack: Magnesium improves blood flow to the heart, prevents blood platelets from clumping together, and stabilizes heart rhythm; magnesium deficiency may increase risk of heart attack and stroke.

Hemorrhoids: Anthocyanins strengthen capillary walls around hemorrhoids and keep tissue from breaking down; fiber helps prevent constipation, which reduces the risk of recurrence.

High cholesterol: Polyphenols and fiber help flush cholesterol from the body.

BLACK BEANS NUTRITION INFORMATION

Serving Size 1 cup black beans, cooked

Amount Per Serving

Calories 227	Calories from fat 8

	% Daily Value*
Total Fat 1 gram	1%
Saturated fat 0 gm	0%
Trans fat 0 gm	†
Cholesterol 0 milligrams	0%
Sodium 2 mg	.08%
Total Carbohydrate 41 gm	14%
Dietary fiber 15 gm	60%
Sugars 0 gm	†
Protein 15 gm	30%
Vitamin A	0%
Vitamin C	0%
Calcium	5%
Iron	20%
Also contains:	
Folate	64%
Manganese	38%
Magnesium	30%
Vitamin B$_1$ (thiamine)	28%
Phosphorus	24%

† Daily Value not established.

* Percent Daily Values are based on a 2,000-calorie diet.

High homocysteine: Folate helps metabolize homocysteine (an amino acid that increases heart-disease risk when levels build up in the blood); low folate levels are associated with high homocysteine levels.

Migraine headache: Magnesium relaxes muscles and nerves and is often low in migraine sufferers.

Obesity: Anthocyanins have been shown to prevent obesity in mice.

Osteo- and rheumatoid arthritis: Anthocyanins reduce inflammation associated with arthritis symptoms.

PMS symptoms: Manganese and magnesium help reduce symptoms, including headache, bloating, and moodiness.

Pregnancy: Folate serves a critical function in growth and reproduction, and protects against a number of congenital malformations, including neural tube birth defects.

Type 2 diabetes: Fiber helps control blood sugar levels after meals by slowing the release of glucose into the bloodstream.

Weight loss and weight control: Fiber-containing foods provide a feeling of fullness; fiber slows digestion, helping to keep blood sugar levels stable and reduce insulin spikes that can trigger cravings and encourage fat storage.

HEALTH SPOTLIGHT

Black Beans Protect Against Cancer

According to research published in *Food Chemistry and Toxicology*, black beans may help guard against cancer. Researchers observed a reduction in the number of pre-cancerous cells in lab animals that were fed a diet containing 20 percent black beans. This was true even with animals that were given a cancer-causing agent. Researchers also tested anthocyanin (an antioxidant compound found in black beans) on its own, but this flavonoid alone actually caused DNA damage. It seems the compounds in black beans work synergistically to reduce pre-cancerous cells.

QUICK TIP

❖ The canning process does not destroy the nutritional value of black beans. Add canned black beans to quesadillas—use whole-wheat tortillas for more protein power.

Black Bean Falafel

YIELD: 3 TO 5 PATTIES

2 15-ounce cans black beans, drained well

1 large egg

$1/2$ cup whole-wheat flour

$1/2$ teaspoon salt

$1/2$ teaspoon black pepper

$1/2$ teaspoon turmeric

$1/2$ teaspoon cayenne pepper

1 teaspoon ground cumin

1 teaspoon ground coriander

3 large whole cloves garlic

$1/4$ cup tightly packed cilantro leaves

2 scallions, green and white parts, roughly chopped

Oil for frying

Put all the ingredients except the oil in the bowl of a food processor. Process on high until mixture is completely smooth. Transfer the mixture to a bowl and refrigerate for at least an hour.

In a large skillet, heat $1/8$ of an inch of vegetable oil—the oil should be hot, but never smoking.

TO FRY FALAFEL BALLS: Use a 1.5- to 2.0-ounce disher, which is like a small ice cream scoop. These are commonly available at restaurant supply stores and gourmet cooking stores. They make it easy because they have a little sweeper that forces the mixture out of the scoop for you. The disher also ensures that each patty will be of equal size and shape. If you don't have a disher, use two large soup spoons. Scoop up the mixture with one spoon and force the mixture off the first spoon with the second spoon.

Gently drop the black bean mixture into the hot skillet in mounds of about two tablespoons. Use the back of a soup spoon to flatten the mound. (Dip the spoon in a little bit of oil so that it won't stick to the top of the mound.) When the patties are golden brown on the first side flip them and cook until golden brown on the second side. Remove cooked patties to a cooling rack positioned over a baking sheet for drainage. Serve hot.

SERVING SUGGESTION: Fill a pita bread halfway with lettuce and diced tomatoes. Add the falafel patties and top with tahini sauce (page 77).

* * *

For other recipes and ways of using black beans, see: Black Bean Burritos with Spicy Chili Salsa (page 77).

12. BLUEBERRIES

"Blueberries is one of the great forces o'good in the world."
—TUMMELER IN *HERE, THERE BE DRAGONS*
BY JAMES A. OWEN, COMIC BOOK ARTIST AND NOVELIST

Native Americans used blueberry juice to treat cough, steeped the leaves to make a tea, and used the fruit as a dye. In fact, it is the deep blue color of these berries that denotes an extremely high antioxidant content. Blueberries rank highest in anti-aging, free-radical destroying antioxidants—beating out sixty other fruits and vegetables—on the ORAC (Oxygen Radical Absorbance Capacity) scale. Especially concentrated are antioxidant anthocyanadins, beneficial in everything from heart disease to varicose veins. And a compound called pterostilbene is as effective as resveratrol (found in red wine) in lowering cholesterol.

HEALTH BENEFITS

Research shows compounds and nutrients found in blueberries may benefit:

Alzheimer's disease: Blueberries improve circulation to the brain and may help slow memory loss (see Health Spotlight).

Cancer: Blueberries contain ellagic acid, an antioxidant compound that blocks metabolic pathways that can lead to cancer.

Cataracts: Anthocyanadins make the walls of blood vessels stronger, helping to deter capillary fragility and improve circulation.

Colon cancer: Eating a diet that includes plenty of blueberries cuts the risk of colon cancer.

Dementia: Anthocyanadins protect the brain from oxidative stress and may benefit symptoms including balance and coordination.

Diarrhea and constipation: Fiber and tannins in blueberries combat both of these conditions simultaneously.

Eye strain: Anthocyanadins increase circulation to the eyes and can be helpful for easing eye strain.

Glaucoma: Anthocyanadins strengthen blood vessel walls, helping to deter capillary fragility and improve circulation.

Heart disease: Pterostilbene was found to be as effective as reservatrol in lowering cholesterol; in one study, blueberries also reduced belly fat, a risk factor for heart disease.

Hemorrhoids: Anthocyanadins strengthen blood vessel walls, helping to deter capillary fragility and improve circulation.

Macular degeneration (age-related): Anthocyanadins help support blood flow to the macula; eating three or more servings of fruit a day may lower risk of macular degeneration.

Night blindness: Bilberries, a blueberry relative, are known for improving World War II pilots' nighttime vision.

BLUEBERRIES NUTRITION INFORMATION		
Serving Size 1 cup blueberries		
Amount Per Serving		
Calories 84	Calories from fat 4	
		% Daily Value
Total Fat 0 grams		0%
Saturated fat 0 gm		1%
Trans fat 0 gm		†
Cholesterol 0 milligrams		0%
Sodium 1 mg		N/A
Total Carbohydrate 21 gm		7%
Dietary fiber 4 gm		14%
Sugars 15 gm		†
Protein 1 gm		2%
Vitamin A		2%
Vitamin C		24%
Calcium		1%
Iron		2%
Also contains:		
Vitamin K		36%
Manganese		25%
† Daily Value not established.		
* Percent Daily Values are based on a 2,000-calorie diet.		

Ovarian cancer: Flavonoids, including kaempferol, guard against ovarian cancer by promoting cancer cell death.

Skin health: Vitamin C aids in collagen formation and protects against free-radical damage, while anthocyanadins enhance the power of vitamin C.

Type 2 diabetes: Eating a diet rich in blueberries has been shown to improve glucose control.

Ulcers: Anthocyanadins may increase the production of stomach mucus and protect the stomach from injury.

Urinary tract infections: Blueberries have the same compounds found in cranberries that help prevent bacteria from adhering to the bladder wall.

Varicose veins: Anthocyanadins strengthen blood vessel walls, helping to deter capillary fragility and development of varicose veins.

HEALTH SPOTLIGHT

Blueberries Are Brain Food

Blueberries could combat Alzheimer's disease. In a study, rats with a genetic tendency toward Alzheimer's disease that were given blueberry extract performed as well as healthy rats in a maze test used to measure cognitive function. Half the rats in the study with the Alzheimer's disease gene (which promotes the buildup of "neuritic plaque" in the brain) were given a diet including blueberry extract for eight months. The other half was fed regular food without blueberry extract. A control group of healthy mice did not receive blueberry extract. All groups were tested for their performance in a maze. The brain-plaqued mice that were fed the blueberry extract performed as well as the healthy control mice—and did much better than the brain-plaqued mice not given the extract. Researchers found increased activity of enzymes called kinases, responsible for cognitive functions including converting short-term to long-term memory, in the brains of the mice fed the blueberry extract.

QUICK TIPS

❖ Power up your yogurt—top plain yogurt (page 217) with blueberries and agave syrup (page 3).

❖ Add blueberries to cereal, muffins, or pancakes; use them as an ice cream topping; or include them in fruit salads—even in green salads.

Blueberry Quick Bread

YIELD: 18 SLICES

$^1/_2$ cup unsweetened soymilk

1 cup Greek-style plain yogurt

$^1/_4$ cup agave nectar

1 egg

$^1/_4$ cup almond butter

2 tablespoons safflower or grape seed oil

$^1/_2$ cup sucanat

1 teaspoon almond extract

1 teaspoon salt

1 cup wheat bran

$^1/_2$ cup rolled oats

$^1/_4$ cup wheat germ

$1^1/_2$ cups whole-wheat flour

1 teaspoon baking powder

1 teaspoon baking soda

2 cups frozen blueberries (do not defrost)

Nonstick cooking spray

Preheat oven to 350°F. Prepare a 9-by-5-inch loaf pan by spraying it with nonstick cooking spray.

In a large bowl, whisk vigorously the soymilk, yogurt, agave nectar, egg, almond butter, oil, sucanat, almond extract, and salt. Set aside for later use.

In a medium bowl, combine well the wheat bran, rolled oats, wheat germ, whole-wheat flour, baking powder, and baking soda. Dump the dry ingredients into the large bowl of wet ingredients. Stir until well combined. Gently fold in the frozen blueberries. Transfer mixture to the prepared loaf pan.

Bake for 60 to 75 minutes, until a toothpick inserted into the center of the loaf comes out with just a few moist crumbs clinging to it. Allow the loaf to cool on a cooling rack in the pan about 10 minutes. Remove it from the pan. Allow it to cool on the cooling rack to room temperature before slicing.

*   *   *

For other recipes and ways of using blueberries, see: Matcha-Blueberry Muesli (page 221).

13. BROCCOLI

This flu season, consider adding more broccoli to your diet. Broccoli contains quercetin, which combats the flu, and is exceptionally high in vitamin C. This cruciferous vegetable has also proven to be a super cancer fighter. Like other cruciferous vegetables such as cauliflower, broccoli contains sulforaphane, a phytonutrient that helps the body detoxify and protects against cancer. Other cancer-fighting compounds in broccoli include the flavonoid kaempferol, associated with a lower risk of ovarian cancer, and indole-3-carbinol, which protects against breast cancer. It's no surprise that broccoli has long held a place in the Mediterranean diet, considered one of the healthiest diets in the world. As early as the fifth century A.D., broccoli was harvested by Roman farmers, who associated the vegetable with one of their revered deities, referring to broccoli as "the five green fingers of Jupiter."

HEALTH BENEFITS

Research shows compounds and nutrients found in broccoli may benefit:

Alzheimer's disease: Eating a diet high in folate was found to lower Alzheimer's risk by half.

Asthma: Quercetin works to prevent immune cells from releasing histamines (chemicals that cause allergic reactions) and may help reduce symptoms such as wheezing.

Bladder cancer: Glucosinolates appear to fight bladder cancer by regulating enzymes that promote the formation of anti-carcinogens.

Breast cancer: Indole-3-carbinole eliminates excess estrogen that can contribute to tumor cell growth in breast tissue.

Cancer: Sulforaphane may help the body detoxify potential carcinogens and protect against cancer.

Cataracts: Lutein and zeaxanthin (two carotenoids found in broccoli as well as in the eye lens) may help slow development.

Colon cancer: Sulforaphane suppresses cell-signaling enyzmes called kinases that promote colon cancer.

Common cold: Vitamin C boosts the immune system to fend off colds and reduce the duration of colds.

Eczema: Quercetin acts like an antihistamine and may help reduce symptoms such as rash and itchy skin.

Flu: Quercetin reduces likelihood of getting the flu.

Gingivitis: Vitamin C promotes healing, especially of bleeding gums.

Hay fever: Quercetin helps prevent immune cells from releasing histamines that trigger allergic symptoms such as itchy, watery eyes and sneezing.

Heart health: Indole-3-carbinol was found to reduce plaque formation in the arteries.

High cholesterol: Fiber reduces cholesterol by binding bile and cholesterol together and helping to shuttle it out of the body.

Immunity: Vitamin C and selenium enhance the immune system's ability to fight infections.

Menstrual cramps: Low levels of calcium can contribute to cramps.

Osteoporosis: Vitamin K helps improve bone density, in part, by slowing calcium loss in bone.

BROCCOLI NUTRITION INFORMATION

Serving Size 1 cup chopped broccoli, raw

Amount Per Serving

Calories 31	Calories from fat 3

	% Daily Value*
Total Fat 0 grams	0%
Saturated fat 0 gm	0%
Trans fat 0 gm	†
Cholesterol 0 milligrams	0%
Sodium 30 mg	1%
Total Carbohydrate 6 gm	2%
Dietary fiber 2 gm	9%
Sugars 2 gm	†
Protein 3 gm	6%
Vitamin A	11%
Vitamin C	135%
Calcium	4%
Iron	4%
Also contains:	
Vitamin K	116%
Folate	14%
Manganese	10%
Vitamin B$_6$ (pyridoxine)	8%

† Daily Value not established.
* Percent Daily Values are based on a 2,000-calorie diet.

Ovarian cancer: Kaempferol may help to suppress ovarian cancer cell growth.

Pregnancy: Folate serves a critical function in growth and reproduction, and protects against a number of congenital malformations, including neural tube birth defects.

Prostate cancer: Just one serving of cruciferous vegetables a week is associated with a 40 percent reduction in prostate tumors.

Skin health: Sulforaphane may help repair sun-damaged skin.

Ulcers: Broccoli helps eliminate *H. pylori* bacteria, which can cause ulcers (see Health Spotlight).

Weight loss and weight control: Fiber-containing foods provide a feeling of fullness; fiber slows digestion, helping to keep blood sugar levels stable and reduce insulin spikes that can trigger cravings and encourage fat storage.

Wrinkles: In a study, women who ate more food containing vitamin C showed fewer wrinkles.

HEALTH SPOTLIGHT

Broccoli Helps Heal Ulcers

A study published in *Inflammopharmacology* found that in people infected with *H. pylori*, a bacteria that causes ulcers, 100 grams (3 ounces) of broccoli sprouts per day resulted in a significant reduction of the bacteria. An *H. pylori* infection is a result of oxidative damage to the cells in the lining of the stomach. In the study, twenty patients infected with *H. pylori* ate broccoli sprouts every day for two months, while twenty patients ate 100 grams of alfalfa sprouts instead. Broccoli sprouts contain about 250 milligrams of sulforaphane glucosinolate per 100 grams, while a serving of alfalfa sprouts contain no sulforaphane glucosinolate. Glucosinolates, naturally occurring compounds in cruciferous vegetables such as broccoli, are converted into sulforaphane when the sprouts are chewed or cut. At the end of the two-month study, subjects who consumed the broccoli sprouts each day showed significantly less *H. pylori*. The alfalfa sprout group showed no change. Researchers speculate that sulforaphane, which can protect against free radicals, contributed to the positive results in the broccoli sprout group.

QUICK TIPS

❖ Keep a bag of finely chopped broccoli in the fridge for a fast addition to quesadillas, quiches or omelets, soups, or baked potatoes. Or add broccoli to brown rice or mix into quinoa in the last minute or two of cooking (page 166).

❖ Dip broccoli florets in anchovy dip (page 14).

Broccoli Lunch Pockets

YIELD: 10 POCKETS

1 8-ounce package frozen filo dough
Olive oil to brush on pastry

Vegetables
$1/4$ cup olive oil
2 large shallots, minced
4 garlic cloves, minced
1 Anaheim chili, seeded and diced
$1 1/2$ pounds broccoli, chopped
(peel stems before chopping)
stems included

Cheese Mixture
8 ounces yogurt
12 ounces beer
$1/4$ cup olive oil
$1/4$ cup flour
Pinch each of salt and pepper
8 ounces sharp cheddar cheese, shredded

Remove the filo dough from the freezer and let it come to room temperature while you prepare the filling.

TO PREPARE THE VEGETABLES: In a large skillet, heat the $1/4$ cup olive oil. Sauté the shallot, garlic, and diced chili until all are soft and fragrant. Add the chopped broccoli and cook just until tender-crisp. Stop as soon as the broccoli takes on a bright color. Set aside.

TO PREPARE THE CHEESE MIXTURE: In a medium bowl, whisk the yogurt and the beer until they are well combined. In a 2-quart saucepan, over low heat, cook the olive oil and flour until the flour is golden and smells nutty (about 3 to 4 minutes). Add the beer/yogurt mixture to the flour/olive oil mixture and whisk vigorously. Add the salt and pepper. Cook over low heat stirring often until the mixture is about the texture of pancake batter. Remove from the heat and immediately stir in the cheese. Continue to stir until the cheese is completely incorporated. In a large bowl, combine the cheese sauce and broccoli. Refrigerate until cool.

TO ASSEMBLE: Preheat oven to 375°F. To assemble each pocket, lay two sheets of filo dough on work surface. One of the short sides of each sheet should be slightly overlapping. Brush the surface of the sheets with a thin layer of olive oil. Fold the sheets in half so that you have one very long strip of dough. Put about 1/3 cup of the cold broccoli mixture at one end of the dough. Use a flag-fold to encase the broccoli creating a triangle. Brush the top of each pocket with additional oil. Bake for 15 to 18 minutes.

* * *

For other recipes and ways of using broccoli, see: Anchovy Quick Tips (page 14).

14. CABBAGE

This humble vegetable, once eaten by the "commoners" of Ireland, is often accompanied by corned beef in the traditional Irish dish. But cabbage has a lot more going for it than we may give it credit for. Like other cruciferous vegetables including broccoli and brussels sprouts, cabbage contains powerful phytonutrients, like kaempferol and indole-3-carbinol, that help our bodies detox and act as formidable cancer fighters. Sulfur compounds called sinigrin activate isothiocyanates, which in turn activate enzymes in the liver that detoxify carcinogens. One of these sulfur compounds even helps to inhibit cell division and stimulate cell death in tumor cells. This could explain why countries like Poland, whose populations eat diets high in cabbage, show lower incidences of cancer than in areas where cabbage is not eaten as frequently.

HEALTH BENEFITS

Research shows compounds and nutrients found in cabbage may benefit:

Alzheimer's disease: Antioxidants, particularly anthocyanins, may protect against the buildup of amyloid beta plaque that results in brain-cell damage.

Asthma: Vitamin C reduces inflammation that can restrict airways.

Bladder cancer: Eating a diet that includes plenty of cruciferous vegetables may cut the risk of bladder cancer by 29 percent.

Breast cancer: Indole-3-carbinol eliminates excess estrogen that can contribute to tumor cell growth in breast tissue.

Colorectal cancer: Sinigrin activates isothiocyanates, which in turn activate enzymes in the liver that eliminate carcinogens and inhibit tumor cell growth in the colon; consuming cruciferous vegetables may cut the risk of colorectal cancer by 49 percent (see Health Spotlight).

Depression: Kaempferol acts as an antidepressant.

Detoxification: Phytonutrients help clear free radicals and toxins.

Gingivitis: Vitamin C promotes healing, especially of bleeding gums.

Heart health: Indole-3-carbinol has been shown to reduce the liver's secretion of apolipoprotein B (the main carrier of harmful LDL cholesterol) by more than half, thus lessening plaque buildup in the arteries.

Immunity: Vitamin C enhances the immune system's ability to fight ear infections, colds, and flu.

Lung cancer: Non-smokers living in a high air-pollution area who regularly ate cruciferous vegetables lowered their lung cancer risk by 30 percent.

Osteo- and rheumatoid arthritis: Vitamin C reduces inflammation and free-radical damage within joints; it is also essential for production and maintenance of collagen, a major protein found in cartilage that helps cushion joints.

CABBAGE NUTRITION INFORMATION		
Serving Size 1 cup chopped red cabbage, fresh		
Amount Per Serving		
Calories 28	Calories from fat 1	
	% Daily Value*	
Total Fat 0 grams	0%	
Saturated fat 0 gm	0%	
Trans fat 0 gm	†	
Cholesterol 0 milligrams	0%	
Sodium 24 mg	1%	
Total Carbohydrate 7 gm	2%	
Dietary fiber 2 gm	7%	
Sugars 3 gm	†	
Protein 1 gm	2%	
Vitamin A	20%	
Vitamin C	85%	
Calcium	4%	
Iron	4%	
Also contains:		
Vitamin K	42%	
Manganese	11%	
† Daily Value not established.		
* Percent Daily Values are based on a 2,000-calorie diet.		

Osteoporosis: Vitamin K helps improve bone density, in part, by slowing calcium loss in bone.

Prostate cancer: Studies show that eating three servings of cruciferous vegetables a week can lower prostate cancer risk by 44 percent.

Skin health: Vitamin C aids in collagen formation and protects against free-radical damage.

Stomach cancer: Cruciferous vegetables are associated with a lower risk of stomach cancer.

Ulcers: Cabbage juice has been shown to heal peptic ulcers.

HEALTH SPOTLIGHT

Cabbage Beat Out Other Vegetables for Cutting Cancer Risk

A study involving more than 100,000 people over a six-year period showed cruciferous vegetables are associated with a much lower risk of cancer. The study, called the Netherlands Cohort Study on Diet and Cancer, showed people who ate vegetables in general had a 25 percent lower risk of colorectal cancers. However, those who ate the most cruciferous vegetables like cabbage, broccoli, and kale, cut their risk by nearly half, showing a 49 percent drop in their colorectal cancer risk.

QUICK TIPS

❖ Use sauerkraut to top burgers and sandwiches. (Sauerkraut has probiotic benefits, too.)

❖ Sauté sliced green cabbage in olive oil, and add salt and freshly ground black pepper to taste. This is a great side or "bed" for fish.

❖ Don't forget the sliced red cabbage in your green salads.

Braised Cabbage Two Ways

Mom's Red Cabbage (Rot Kohl)

YIELD: 4–6 SERVINGS

3 Granny Smith apples, unpeeled, quartered, cored, and thinly sliced

2 cups water

4 tablespoons unsalted butter

$1/8$ teaspoon ground cloves

$3/4$ cup thawed apple juice concentrate

$1/4$ cup red wine vinegar

$1 1/2$ teaspoons kosher salt

2 pounds red cabbage, cored and thinly sliced

In a large skillet combine the apples, water, butter, and cloves. Simmer over medium heat until the apples are soft, about 10 minutes. Add the apple juice concentrate, vinegar, salt, and cabbage. Continue to cook over medium heat, stirring frequently, until the cabbage is soft and the liquid is evaporated.

Dad's Braised Green Cabbage

YIELD: 4–6 SERVINGS

4 tablespoons unsalted butter

1 large brown onion, thinly sliced

$1/_2$ teaspoon ground black pepper

2 pounds green cabbage, thinly sliced

2 cups canned chicken stock

In a large skillet, melt the butter. Sauté the onions until they are soft. Add the chicken stock, pepper, and cabbage. Continue to cook, stirring frequently, until the cabbage is soft and most of the liquid has evaporated.

15. CARROTS

"Vegetables are a must on a diet. I suggest carrot cake,
zucchini bread, and pumpkin pie."
—JIM DAVIS, CARTOONIST
AND CREATOR OF "GARFIELD"

A pleasing paradox was observed in a study when carrot cake was found to keep blood glucose levels steady in diabetics despite its sugar content. The reason for this was not determined by researchers, but our theory is that this phenomena could possibly be attributed to the blood-sugar regulating effects of the carotenoids in carrots. Carrots have been a food and medicine since ancient times, although the Greeks and Romans were familiar only with white and purple varieties. Today, red, purple, yellow, white, and orange carrots are cultivated around the world, each containing a slightly different array of phytonutrients. The orange variety that we know and love, however, is actually the richest source of vitamin A carotenes of any vegetable. This pancakes recipe—with a hint of orange, and drizzled with cream cheese and lime icing—is a great way to eat your carrots.

HEALTH BENEFITS

Research shows compounds and nutrients found in carrots may benefit:

Bladder cancer: Eating a diet rich in carotenoid-containing foods may lower risk of this cancer by 50 percent.

Brain health: Beta-carotene was shown to protect against cognitive decline.

Breast cancer: Eating a diet that includes plenty of carotenoid-containing foods may cut breast cancer risk after menopause by 20 percent.

Cancer (cervical, laryngeal, prostate, and esophageal cancers): Carotenoids have been linked to decreased risk.

Colon cancer: The phytonutrient falcrinol, which acts as a fungicide, may be responsible for warding off this type of cancer.

Digestive health: Fiber improves digestion and is linked to a reduced risk of hemorrhoids and diverticulitis (bulging tissue pouches in the colon).

Heart disease: Carotenoid-rich foods including carrots and squash eaten daily reduced risk of heart attack by 60 percent in one study.

High cholesterol: Fiber reduces cholesterol by binding bile and blood cholesterol together and helping to shuttle it out of the body.

Lung health: Vitamin A helps repair the lining of the respiratory tract and may guard against infection and damage from smoking or secondhand smoke.

Night blindness: Vitamin A is converted to rhodopsin, a protein in the retina that is responsible for night vision.

**CARROTS
NUTRITION INFORMATION**

Serving Size 1 cup chopped carrots, raw

Amount Per Serving

Calories 52	Calories from fat 3
	% Daily Value*
Total Fat 0 grams	0%
Saturated fat 0 gm	0%
Trans fat 0 gm	†
Cholesterol 0 milligrams	0%
Sodium 88 mg	4%
Total Carbohydrate 12 gm	4%
Dietary fiber 4 gm	14%
Sugars 6 gm	†
Protein 1 gm	2%
Vitamin A	428%
Vitamin C	13%
Calcium	4%
Iron	2%
Also contains:	
Vitamin K	21%
Potassium	12%
Manganese	9%

Carrots are also a good source of fiber, vitamin B_1 (thiamine), vitamin B_3 (niacin), vitamin B_6 (pyridoxine), and folate.

† Daily Value not established.
* Percent Daily Values are based on a 2,000-calorie diet.

Osteoporosis: Vitamin K helps improve bone density, in part, by slowing calcium loss in bone.

Type 2 diabetes: A high intake of carotenoid-rich foods is associated with lower blood sugar levels.

HEALTH SPOTLIGHT

Can Carrots Make You More Attractive?

Although the jury is still out for humans, beta-carotene, abundant in carrots, appears to do just that in fish. A study of male fish revealed that those whose diets were supplemented with beta-carotene increased their appeal to the female species by making their bodies more colorful and attractive, and signifying adequate health necessary to care for offspring. The carotenoids also enhanced their immunity and helped them live longer because their bodies were better able to combat oxidative stress.

QUICK TIP

❖ Buy pre-shredded carrots to keep on hand to add to wraps and pitas, layer in lasagna, or toss into salads.

Carrot Griddle Cakes with Cream Cheese Topping

YIELD: 4 SERVINGS (2 cakes each)

Topping
4 ounces cream cheese, at room temperature

$1/4$ cup honey

2 tablespoons thawed apple juice concentrate

1–2 tablespoons fresh lime juice
(more or less to taste)

1 teaspoon vanilla

Zest of 1 lime (zest before juicing)

Cakes
2 cups whole-wheat flour

$1/2$ cups dried, unsweetened coconut

2 teaspoons baking powder

1 teaspoon cinnamon

1 teaspoon ground ginger

1 teaspoon nutmeg

$^1/_8$ teaspoon ground cloves

$^1/_4$ teaspoon salt

3 eggs beaten well

$^3/_4$ cup apple juice concentrate

1 cup coconut milk

1 teaspoon vanilla extract

2 cups grated carrots

Vegetable oil for griddle

TO MAKE THE TOPPING: In the bowl of a stand mixer or with a hand mixer, beat the cream cheese until soft. Slowly add the honey, mixing well to combine. Do the same with the apple juice concentrate and lime juice. Stir in the vanilla and zest. Refrigerate until you are ready to serve the griddle cakes.

TO MAKE THE CAKES: In a large mixing bowl, combine the flour, coconut, baking powder, spices, and salt. In a medium mixing bowl, combine the eggs, apple juice concentrate, coconut milk, vanilla, and carrots. Pour the wet ingredients into the dry ingredients and mix well. Prepare the griddle with a thin coat of vegetable oil, and heat over a low heat. Keeping the griddle at a low heat, ladle about $^1/_4$ cup of the batter onto the skillet to make a griddle cake. Cook until bubbles break the surface of the pancakes, edges start to look dry, and the undersides are golden brown, about 4 minutes. Flip with a spatula and cook about 2 more minutes on the second side. Repeat with the remaining batter, adding more oil to the skillet as needed.

Drizzle the cakes with the cream cheese topping and serve.

* * *

For other recipes and ways of using carrots, see: Apricot Moroccan-Style Stew (page 23) Millet Hash (page 129), Tomato-Seafood Chowder (page 203).

16. CHERRIES

After Mount Vesuvius erupted in 79 B.C., destroying the nearby village of Pompeii, among the foods found in the remains were cherries. Cherries are still a popular fruit of the Mediterranean. Today, science has discovered that cherries contain powerful antioxidants known as anthocyanins, plus bioflavonoids that inhibit COX-1 and COX-2 inflammatories to reduce arthritis pain, quercetin (a flavonoid that can fend off the flu), and ellagic acid (an anticarcinogen that can inhibit cancer). Additionally, melatonin, a hormone linked to enhanced sleep and reduced depression, is found in high amounts in cherries. Antioxidants are especially concentrated in dried cherries, ranking higher on the ORAC scale than fresh cherries. However, fresh cherries, both tart and sweet, are also excellent sources, along with tart cherry juice.

HEALTH BENEFITS

Research shows compounds and nutrients found in cherries may benefit:

Belly fat: Research shows tart cherries may help reduce belly fat, a diabetes risk factor.

Brain health: Antioxidants, particularly anthocyanins, may protect brain cells from oxidative damage.

Breast cancer: Melatonin appears to slow the growth of breast cancer.

Colon cancer: Anthocyanins were found to slow cancer cell growth.

Depression: Melatonin has shown benefit in relieving depression, especially postmenopausal depression.

Flu: Quercetin reduces the likelihood of getting the flu.

Gout and gout pain: Cherries reduce the formation of painful uric acid crystals in the joints and may decrease frequency of future attacks.

Heart health: Anthocyanins act as anti-inflammatories that protect the heart.

High blood pressure: Ellagic acid may help reduce blood pressure.

High cholesterol: Powdered cherries lowered cholesterol in a study.

Insomnia: Melatonin induces relaxation and sleep.

Jet lag: Melatonin may help the body's internal clock adjust to a new time zone.

Osteo- and rheumatoid arthritis: Anthocyanins may ease inflammation and reduce arthritis-related pain.

Post-workout muscle pain: Cherry juice was found to relieve exercise-induced pain (see Health Spotlight).

Prostate cancer: Ellagic acid may inhibit proliferation of cancer cells.

Type 2 diabetes: Anthocyanins have been shown to help lower blood sugar levels in people with diabetes.

CHERRIES NUTRITION INFORMATION

Serving Size 1 cup sour cherries, fresh

Amount Per Serving

Calories 77	Calories from fat 4

	% Daily Value*
Total Fat 0 grams	0%
Saturated fat 0 gm	0%
Trans fat 0 gm	†
Cholesterol 0 milligrams	0%
Sodium 5 mg	.2%
Total Carbohydrate 19 gm	6%
Dietary fiber 2 gm	10%
Sugars 13 gm	†
Protein 2 gm	4%
Vitamin A	40%
Vitamin C	26%
Calcium	2%
Iron	3%
Also contains:	
Manganese	9%
Potassium	8%

† Daily Value not established.
* Percent Daily Values are based on a 2,000-calorie diet.

HEALTH SPOTLIGHT

Ease Muscle Pain with Cherry Juice

Anti-inflammatories in cherry juice were shown to alleviate muscle pain from exercise in a study. Study participants drank either 12 ounces of a cherry juice blend, containing the equivalent of about fifty tart cherries, twice a day, for three days before exercise and for four days afterward, or a placebo juice. After performing muscle-damaging exercise, tests showed the average pain score was significantly less in those drinking the cherry juice. Additionally, pain peaked at twenty-four hours for those drinking cherry juice, but continued to increase for forty-eight hours for those on the placebo juice.

QUICK TIPS

❖ Add dried cherries to trail mix, granola, or oatmeal (page 136).

❖ Make an easy chicken salad by mixing chopped roasted chicken with mayo and dried cherries.

❖ Add frozen cherries to smoothies.

Cherry-Aki Salmon with Cherry-Studded Quinoa

YIELD: 4 SERVINGS

Quinoa

3 cups water

2 tablespoons soy sauce

$1^1/_2$ cups quinoa

1 teaspoon ground ginger

6 ounces dried cherries

Cherry Sauce

4 cups black cherry juice (not tart)

2 cups pineapple juice

$^1/_4$ cup honey

2 tablespoons soy sauce

3 cloves garlic, minced

2 tablespoons fresh ginger, minced

Salmon

2 cups whole-grain flake cereal, crushed into fine crumbs
$2/3$ cup finely minced walnuts
1 tablespoon ground ginger
1 teaspoon each kosher salt and ground pepper
1 cup whole-wheat flour
2 eggs, beaten well
4 boneless, skinless salmon fillets (6 ounces each)
$1/4$ cup olive oil

TO COOK THE QUINOA: Bring the water and soy sauce to a boil. Add the quinoa, ginger, and cherries. Stir. Bring back up to a boil. Reduce the heat to low. Cook covered for about 15 minutes, until all the water is absorbed. Check and stir frequently.

TO MAKE THE SAUCE: Combine all the ingredients for the sauce in a large pan. Over low heat, reduce the sauce to $1/3$ of its original volume (about 2 cups). Stir frequently. Meanwhile, prepare the rest of the meal.

TO COOK THE FISH: Combine the cereal, walnuts, ginger, and salt and pepper. Set up your dredging station as follows: flour in one shallow dish, eggs in a second shallow dish, and cereal mix in a third. Dredge each fillet in the flour to completely coat, then dip it in the eggs. Gently press each side of each fillet into the cereal mixture. Heat the oil in a large skillet. Transfer the fillets to the hot skillet. Cook each fillet 3 to 4 minutes per side. To plate the meal, place a piece of fish over a serving of quinoa. Cover the fish and quinoa with the cherry sauce.

*   *   *

For other recipes and ways of using cherries, see: Stuffed Date Appetizer with Pomegranate Dipping Sauce (page 96), Strawberry Summer Pudding (page 195), Almond-Cherry Muesli (page 220).

17. CHILI PEPPERS

They spice up Texas chili, add heat to hot sauces, and even give some chocolate confections a kick. There are entire conventions, cookoffs, and festivals devoted to the chili pepper. Chili pepper fans seem to instinctively know that this fiery food and spice not only wakes up the taste buds, but there's just something about it that makes them feel good. It turns out chili peppers, both fresh and dried, contain capsaicin, a phytochemical that stimulates the body's natural pain-killing endorphins, releasing powerful feel-good chemicals in the body. The hotter the pepper, the greater the capsaicin content. But aside from their endorphin-stimulating abilities, chilies are also incredibly rich in vitamins A and C (a single Anaheim chili, for example, packs 170 percent of the Daily Value of vitamin A and 80 percent of vitamin C). Plus, they contain carotenoids including lutein and zeaxanthin. While the recipe here uses the green Anaheim variety, also check out the recipes on pages 156 and 200 that use pasilla and chipotle chilies.

HEALTH BENEFITS

Research shows compounds and nutrients found in chilies may benefit:

Allergies: Vitamin C reduces inflammation associated with allergy symptoms.

Asthma: Capsaicin stimulates secretions that help clear mucus congestion from the lungs.

Atherosclerosis: Antioxidants decrease the oxidation of harmful LDL cholesterol (see Health Spotlight); eating a diet rich in carotenoids can lower the risk of atherosclerosis.

Cataracts: Vitamin A-containing foods are effective in reducing risk of cataracts.

Cluster headaches: Capsaicin's pain-relieving properties help alleviate headaches.

Gout: In one study, vitamin C intake was shown to cut risk as much as 45 percent.

Chili Peppers

Immunity: Vitamin A helps keep skin and mucous membranes that line the nose, sinuses, and mouth healthy and protects against invading pathogens; vitamin C enhances the immune system's ability to fight ear infections, colds, and flu.

Inflammation: Capsaicin reduces the inflammation response, possibly by inhibiting substance P, a protein involved with triggering inflammation.

Leukemia: Capsaicin inhibits the growth of adult T-cell leukemia cells, a type of leukemia resistant to conventional chemotherapy.

Lung cancer: Foods rich in beta-carotene may provide protection against lung cancer.

Macular degeneration (age-related): Lutein and zeaxanthin help retain macular pigments in the eye and antioxidants reduce free-radical damage.

Osteo- and rheumatoid arthritis: Capsaicin causes the brain to secrete more pain-killing endorphins.

Osteoporosis: Vitamin C slows bone loss.

Prostate cancer: In one study, capsaicin significantly reduced the growth and the size of prostate tumors.

Type 2 diabetes: Increased consumption of capsaicin-containing foods may help reduce the amount of insulin required to lower blood sugar after a meal.

Ulcers: Capsaicin helps kill *H. pylori* bacteria, which cause peptic ulcers, while activating stomach cells to secrete protective buffering juices.

CHILI PEPPERS NUTRITION INFORMATION

Serving Size 1 Anaheim chili

Amount Per Serving

Calories 20	Calories from fat 0

	% Daily Value
Total Fat 0 grams	0%
Saturated fat 0 gm	0%
Trans fat 0 gm	†
Cholesterol 0 milligrams	0%
Sodium 10 mg	.4%
Total Carbohydrate 3 gm	1%
Dietary fiber 0 gm	0%
Sugars 2 gm	†
Protein 1 gm	2%
Vitamin A	80%
Vitamin C	170%
Calcium	0%
Iron	0%

† Daily Value not established.
* Percent Daily Values are based on a 2,000-calorie diet.

Weight control and weight loss: The heat in chili peppers raises thermogenesis (heat production) and oxygen consumption in the body, which in turn increases metabolism and helps burn calories.

HEALTH SPOTLIGHT

Red Chilies Good for the Heart

A study published in the *British Journal of Nutrition* concludes that eating freshly chopped red chili peppers may protect blood fats such as cholesterol and triglycerides from free-radical damage that can lead to atherosclerosis. The study examined a group of twenty-seven people who ate either 1 ounce of fresh red peppers including cayenne a day, or no chilies, for a month. The results showed that free-radical damage was significantly lower in those on the chili-pepper diet. In males who consumed the chilies, a lower resting heart rate was seen, as well as a greater amount of blood reaching the heart.

QUICK TIPS

❖ Add a pinch of cayenne pepper to a cup of hot cocoa.

❖ Add diced chilies to guacamole and omelets.

❖ Top burgers or grilled chicken with roasted green chilies such as Anaheim, poblano, or hatch. Pair with Monterey Jack cheese if desired—the flavors complement each other.

Black Bean Burritos with Spicy Chili Salsa

YIELD: 6 BURRITOS

Chili Salsa

1 pound fresh Anaheim chilies or a combination
of chilies such as poblano and Anaheim, roasted
(directions to roast chilies follow)

2 scallions, green and white parts, thinly sliced

$1/2$ cup loosely packed cilantro leaves,
coarsely chopped

1 avocado, diced small

$1/2$ cup plain Greek-style yogurt

2 tablespoons fresh squeezed lime juice,
or more to taste

Zest from squeezed limes (zest before juicing)

Salt and pepper to taste

Bean Filling

2 15-ounce cans black beans

2 tablespoons safflower oil

1 small onion, diced (about 1 cup)

3 cloves garlic, minced

1 cup homemade or canned chicken stock

1 to 3 teaspoons minced chipotle in adobo
(more or less, depending on your tolerance for heat)

$1/2$ teaspoon salt

6 10-inch whole-grain tortillas

TO MAKE THE SALSA: Begin by roasting the chilies (see the inset on the following page). When they are cool, dice gently and combine the chilies, scallions, cilantro, avocado, yogurt, lime juice, and zest. Season with salt and pepper to taste. Store in the refrigerator until you are ready to serve.

TO MAKE THE BEAN FILLING: Drain the liquid from both cans of beans. In a food processor or blender, puree one can of the black beans. Leave the other can whole. Heat the oil in a 2-quart saucepan over medium heat. Add the onions, sautéing until soft, about 3 minutes. Add the garlic and cook about 2 minutes longer. Add the chicken stock, whole

---

Roasting Chili Peppers

To roast chili peppers (or any other type of pepper), hold the chilies, one by one, above the flame of a gas burner and allow the skin to char. Use tongs to hold the chilies—don't use a kitchen fork, as it can be difficult to get the chilies off the fork safely when they're hot. Once you have blackened the skin on one side, turn to expose more green skin to the flame. Once all of the skin has been blackened, put the chilies in a casserole dish and cover tightly with plastic wrap. This will allow it to steam. Repeat this process with each chili, adding the charred chilies to the casserole, one by one, and covering. When you have finished with the last of the chilies, allow them to sit, covered, continuing to steam for about 5 minutes. Next, run the chilies under cold water to wash away the charred skin. Remove the stems and seeds, but leave as much of the membrane as possible. (The membrane is where the bulk of the capsaicin is found.) If you don't have a gas stove, roast the chilies in a preheated 350°F oven for 3 to 5 minutes, or until they puff up. Steam and remove skins as described above.

---

beans, chipotle chili, and salt. Whisk in the pureed beans. Continue to cook over a medium-low flame, stirring frequently, for about 20 minutes, until the beans are the texture of refried beans.

To serve, warm the tortillas. Spoon one-sixth of the beans and the chili salsa in the center of each tortilla and roll up gently.

*   *   *

For other recipes and ways of using chili peppers, see: Coffee-Braised Pork Loin (page 82), Pineapple Salsa on Shrimp Patties (page 155), Smoky Sweet Potatoes (page 200).

18. COFFEE

*"If it weren't for the coffee, I'd have
no identifiable personality whatsoever."*
—DAVID LETTERMAN

We love our morning jolt of java, but may feel a twinge of guilt. Isn't caffeine supposed to be bad for us? There are so many conflicting reports, what are we to believe? Here's the good news. Aside from caffeine (which, as it turns out, isn't all bad), coffee is also chock-full of antioxidants including chlorogenic acid and tocopherols, and beneficial compounds such as quinines that increase insulin sensitivity and may cut your risk of developing type 2 diabetes. Coffee also contains the mineral magnesium, which could explain its benefits in headache relief and possibly PMS. And although coffee has been known to stain teeth, it contains trigonelline, which is antibacterial and can prevent cavities! So as long as you don't overdo it, which could lead to problems like nervousness and rapid heartbeat, experts say coffee is okay, even beneficial.

HEALTH BENEFITS

Research shows compounds and nutrients found in coffee may benefit:

Alertness: Caffeine proved to boost alertness in controlled studies.

Alzheimer's disease: Coffee may help protect against the buildup of amyloid beta plaque that results in brain-cell damage.

Asthma: People who drink coffee regularly have one-third fewer asthmatic symptoms than non-coffee drinkers, perhaps due to the caffeine, which helps relax airways.

Athletic endurance and performance: Caffeine enhances exercise performance, perhaps by increasing adrenaline levels.

Cavities: Trigonelline's antibacterial and anti-adhesive properties have been shown to prevent dental cavities from forming.

Cognitive performance: Caffeine improves alertness, which can boost concentration.

Colon cancer: Three or more cups a day may reduce colon cancer risk in women by half.

Concentration: Caffeine was found to improve concentration in night-shift workers.

Depression: Coffee lifts mood and is associated with lower rates of suicide.

Erectile dysfunction: Caffeine, a vasodilator, may help men with diabetes overcome erectile dys-function.

Gallstones: Men who drank three cups daily had nearly half the risk of developing gallstones of non-coffee drinkers.

Heart disease: Drinking one to three cups of coffee daily appears to protect women from heart disease.

Libido: Coffee may increase desire (see Health Spotlight).

COFFEE NUTRITION INFORMATION

Serving Size 8 ounces (1 cup) coffee, brewed

Amount Per Serving

Calories 2	Calories from fat 0

	% Daily Value*
Total Fat 0 grams	0%
Saturated fat 0 gm	0%
Trans fat 0 gm	†
Cholesterol 0 milligrams	0%
Sodium 5 mg	.2%
Total Carbohydrate 0 gm	0%
Dietary fiber 0 gm	0%
Sugars 0 gm	†
Protein 0 gm	0%
Vitamin A	0%
Vitamin C	0%
Calcium	0%
Iron	0%
Also contains:	
Vitamin B$_2$ (riboflavin)	11%
Manganese	3%
Magnesium	2%
Phosphorus	1%

† Daily Value not established.

* Percent Daily Values are based on a 2,000-calorie diet.

Life expectancy: Coffee drinkers have slightly lower mortality rates than non-coffee drinkers.

Liver disease: Coffee benefits hepatitis C and lowers the risk of cirrhosis in heavy drinkers by 22 percent.

Metabolism: Caffeine may increase metabolic rate.

Migraine headache: Riboflavin and magnesium may reduce the frequency of migraine attacks.

Muscle soreness: Caffeine can ease pain related to exercise.

Parkinson's disease: One study showed people who drank coffee were five times less likely to develop the disease, possibly due to increasing the amount of depleted dopamine (a neurotransmitter) in the brain.

PMS symptoms: Magnesium and manganese help relieve symptoms, including mood swings, bloating, and headaches.

Type 2 diabetes: Quinines, chlorogenic acid, and tocopherols, plus magnesium have been shown to improve insulin sensitivity and glucose metabolism.

HEALTH SPOTLIGHT

A Libation That Enhances Libido?

A cup of coffee may increase your sex drive, according to a study published in the journal *Pharmacology Biochemistry and Behavior.* Female rats that were given a dose of caffeine equivalent to a cup of coffee thirty minutes before mating were more amorous than those that were given more or less caffeine.

QUICK TIPS

❖ Add a dash of cinnamon to coffee grounds before brewing.

❖ For iced coffee that doesn't taste watered down, make coffee ice cubes: freeze coffee in an ice cube tray and use in place of ice.

❖ Consider choosing regular over decaffeinated. In one Harvard study, subjects drinking decaf coffee showed a reduced diabetes risk, but only half that of those drinking caffeinated coffee. Some benefits, such as increased alertness and muscle endurance, are attributed to coffee's caffeine content.

Coffee-Braised Pork Loin

YIELD: 8 SERVINGS

3 cups hot, very strong coffee

1 firmly packed cup golden raisins

2 to 3 dried ancho chilies

(depending on your tolerance for heat)

4 pounds pork loin*

Salt and pepper

$1/_4$ cup safflower oil

1 large brown onion, thinly sliced

$1/_4$ cup fresh squeezed lime juice

8 ounces canned tomato sauce

$1/_2$ heaping teaspoon cinnamon

$1/_2$ heaping teaspoon cumin

1 heaping teaspoon dried, crushed oregano leaves

1 vanilla bean, split lengthwise

Finely grated zest from squeezed limes

(zest before juicing)

*For a more traditional braise, you can use the shoulder butt cut. This cut can be a little too fatty, but if you use it, trim and discard the excess fat from the surface of the roast before you begin.

Preheat oven to 300°F.

In a small bowl, soak the raisins in $1^1/_2$ cups of the hot coffee. Set aside for later use. In another small bowl, soak the ancho chilies in the other $1^1/_2$ cups of hot coffee. Set aside for later use.

Pat the surface of the roast dry with paper towels. Liberally salt and pepper the entire surface of the roast. In the bottom of a large Dutch oven, heat the safflower oil on high until you see ripples on the surface. Place the roast in the hot oil and allow a brown crust to form before turning. Turn the roast three times to obtain a brown crust on each side. Turn only once the crust has had time to form. Remove the roast from the pan and set aside.

Turn the flame down to very low and add the sliced onion to the oil left in the pan. Use a spoon to scrape loose any fond (brown carmelized bits from the roast) that has formed on the bottom of the pan. Allow the onions to caramelize over very low heat stirring infrequently, until they take on a golden brown color.

In the meantime, remove the chilies from the coffee in which they have been soaking. Do not discard the soaking liquid. Remove and discard the chili stems. Extricate and discard the seeds. Run the soaking liquid through a sieve to remove any seeds. In the jar of a blender, combine the cleaned chilies with their soaking liquid, the raisins with their soaking liquid, the lime juice, tomato sauce, cinnamon, cumin, and oregano. Blend on high until you have a completely smooth sauce.

Once onions have been caramelized, return the roast and any juices that may have accumulated to the Dutch oven. Pour the coffee sauce over the roast. Add the whole vanilla bean to the sauce. Cover and place Dutch oven in the oven. Braise 3 hours. Turn the roast once an hour.

Remove the Dutch oven from the oven and shred the meat. Remove vanilla bean from sauce. Return the shredded meat to the sauce and return the Dutch oven, uncovered, to the oven for another 30 minutes to thicken the sauce. Stir in the zest. Serve over rice, or as part of a tostada on a corn tortilla with beans and guacamole.

* * *

For other recipes and ways of using coffee, see: Agave Quick Tips (page 5), Coffee-Coconut Muesli (page 221).

19. CUCUMBERS

Cucumber slices are often applied over the eyes during facials because they decrease puffiness. It is the ascorbic acid (vitamin C) and the antioxidant caffeic acid in cucumbers that reduce water retention. The ancient Egyptians knew this and used cucumber for both the skin and as a food. (Perhaps this is what helped Cleopatra look so beautiful.) Also contributing to radiant skin is silica, a component of connective tissue. And cucumbers contain the trace mineral molybdenum, which may benefit asthma, along with tryptophan, an amino acid that promotes relaxation. In fact, it could be cucumber's ability to help relax you, as well as cool you off in summer salads, that inspired the expression "cool as a cucumber."

HEALTH BENEFITS

Research shows compounds and nutrients found in cucumbers may benefit:

Alzheimer's disease: Silica may mitigate harmful effects of aluminum on the brain.

Anxiety: Tryptophan is necessary for the synthesis of the feel-good chemical serotonin that helps regulate anxiety and mood.

Asthma: Molybdenum helps to detoxify sulfites related to asthma attacks.

Dental Health: Molybdenum is required for tooth enamel.

Digestive health: Fiber along with cucumber's high water content (about 95 percent) work to keep digestion running smoothly.

Healthy hair, skin, and nails: Silica and vitamin C help form the connective tissue that gives skin, hair, and nails their strength and elasticity.

High blood pressure: In one study, foods high in potassium, magnesium, and fiber lowered blood pressure to healthier levels and decreased risk of stroke.

Cucumbers

Insomnia: Tryptophan is a precursor for serotonin, a neurotransmitter that regulates sleep.

Irritable bowel syndrome: Soluble fiber benefits symptoms including gas, pain, and bloating.

Muscle soreness: Silica and vitamin C are essential components of healthy connective tissue including muscle; research has shown that vitamin C, which also acts as an anti-inflammatory, decreases delayed-onset muscle soreness.

Osteo- and rheumatoid arthritis: Silica works with calcium to strengthen bone, and with vitamin C to form collagen (a major protein found in cartilage that helps cushion joints); vitamin C limits free-radical damage and inflammation.

Osteoporosis: Silicon, calcium, manganese, and vitamin K are important for building bone and preventing bone loss and fractures (see Health Spotlight).

Skin irritations: Caffeic acid reduces swelling.

CUCUMBERS NUTRITION INFORMATION	
Serving Size 1/2 cup sliced cucumber, with skin	
Amount Per Serving	
Calories 8	Calories from fat 0
	% Daily Value*
Total Fat 0 grams	0%
Saturated fat 0 gm	0%
Trans fat 0 gm	†
Cholesterol 0 milligrams	0%
Sodium 1 mg	.04%
Total Carbohydrate 2 gm	1%
Dietary fiber .3 gm	1%
Sugars 1 gm	†
Protein 0 gm	0%
Vitamin A	1%
Vitamin C	2%
Calcium	1%
Iron	1%
Also contains:	
Vitamin K	11%
Potassium	2%
Magnesium	2%
Manganese	2%
Folate	1%
† Daily Value not established.	
* Percent Daily Values are based on a 2,000-calorie diet.	

Weight loss and weight control: Fiber-containing foods provide a feeling of fullness; fiber slows digestion, helping to keep blood sugar levels stable and reduce insulin spikes that can trigger cravings and encourage fat storage.

HEALTH SPOTLIGHT

Cucumbers May Benefit Osteoporosis

Silica, or silicon dioxide, a macromineral found in abundance in cucumbers, may be essential to keeping bones strong. Researchers gave silicon to a group of women with osteoporosis or osteopenia (bone density less than normal). The women took 3, 6, or 12 milligrams of silicon in addition to supplementing with calcium and vitamin D. Over the course of a year, significant improvements in bone turnover (breaking down of old bone and formation of new bone) as well as bone collagen were seen in the femurs of the women taking either 6 or 12 milligrams of silicon compared to those taking only calcium and vitamin D.

QUICK TIPS

❖ Cucumber juice promotes a glowing, healthy complexion, and helps strengthen nails and hair. Use a juicer to juice fresh cucumbers.

❖ Add cucumber slices to water or other cold beverages for a crisp and refreshing drink.

Cucumber Relish

YIELD: 6 SERVINGS

2 teaspoons anchovy paste

$^1/_4$ cup safflower or canola mayonnaise

$^3/_4$ cup Greek-style yogurt

2 scallions, green and white parts, minced

2 tablespoons minced flat leaf parsley

2 teaspoons minced tarragon leaves

1 teaspoon minced basil

1 tablespoon minced shallots

2 tablespoons fresh squeezed lemon juice

Zest from lemon (zest before juicing)

2 cups cucumber, diced small

Salt to taste

In the bowl of a food processor, combine the anchovy paste, mayonnaise, yogurt, scallions, parsley, tarragon, basil, shallots, lemon juice, and lemon zest. Process on high until you have a smooth dressing. Transfer dressing to a large bowl. Toss the cucumber in the dressing to evenly coat. Serve over grilled fish or with pita chips as an appetizer.

20. DARK CHOCOLATE

"If you are not feeling well, if you have not slept,
chocolate will revive you. But you have no chocolate!
My dear, how will you ever manage?"
—MARQUISE DE SÉVIGNÉ, A FRENCH ARISTOCRAT (1626–1698),
IN A LETTER TO A FRIEND

For chocolate lovers who have long believed in chocolate's therapeutic powers, research discovering its health benefits just confirmed what they suspected all along. "Chemically speaking, chocolate really is the world's perfect food," states Michael Levine, nutrition researcher, in his book *The Emperors of Chocolate: Inside the Secret World of Hershey and Mars* (San Val, 2001). All in all, there are about 300 chemicals in chocolate, some of which appear to increase serotonin to lift mood and fight depression, trigger endorphins to alleviate pain, increase sexual function and desire, and reduce stress. Dark chocolate is high in antioxidants including epicatechin, a powerful flavonoid, and other flavonoids including procyanidins and catechins, which appear to help give chocolate health-promoting powers to those normally attributed to fruits and vegetables. Chocolate also contains minerals, including magnesium and calcium (both shown to fight symptoms of PMS), as well as potassium. Some claim just the aroma of chocolate alone can alter brain waves to induce relaxation. And although chocolate bars contain fat, the fat content in high-quality chocolate bars is about one-third oleic acid, which is unsaturated and found in olive oil, and one-third stearic acid and one-third palmitic oil, which are saturated, but do not appear to raise cholesterol.

HEALTH BENEFITS

Research shows compounds and nutrients found in chocolate may benefit:

Blood clots: Cocoa flavonoids have an aspirin-like effect on blood platelets, making them less likely to clot.

Blood vessel function: Epicatechins trigger substances that increase blood flow in arteries.

Cancer: Epicatechins stopped breast cancer cells from dividing in one study.

Chronic fatigue syndrome: Polyphenols in chocolate were found to lessen fatigue.

Cognitive function: Epicatechins are thought to improve memory, presumably by improving blood flow to the brain.

Coughs: A chocolate chemical called theobromine functions as a cough suppressant and in one study was found to be more effective than codeine.

Diarrhea: Cocoa flavonoids bind to a protein in the intestines that regulates fluid secretion.

Heart attack: Research links chocolate to reduced risk (see Health Spotlight).

High blood pressure: Potassium and cocoa flavonoids appear to lower blood pressure, possibly by improving flexibility of blood vessels.

DARK CHOCOLATE NUTRITION INFORMATION

Serving Size 1 ounce (28 grams) dark chocolate, 70–85% cacao solids

Amount Per Serving

Calories 168   Calories from fat 108

	% Daily Value*
Total Fat 12 grams	18%
Saturated fat 7.1 gm	35%
Trans fat 0 gm	†
Cholesterol 1 milligram	.1%
Sodium 6 mg	.2%
Total Carbohydrate 13 gm	4%
Dietary fiber 3 gm	12%
Sugars 7 gm	†
Protein 2 gm	3.5%
Vitamin A	0%
Vitamin C	0%
Calcium	2%
Iron	19%
Also contains:	
Copper	25%
Manganese	27%
Magnesium	16%
Potassium	6%

Note: Pure cocoa powder contains minimal sugars.
† Daily Value not established.
* Percent Daily Values are based on a 2,000-calorie diet.

High cholesterol: Cocoa flavonoids lower LDL (bad) cholesterol levels by increasing antioxidant activity in the blood.

Life expectancy: Eating a diet that includes plenty of cocoa-rich foods is associated with a reduced risk of death from heart attack and stroke.

PMS symptoms: Magnesium and calcium help relieve symptoms including headache, bloating, and moodiness.

Tooth decay: Cocoa contains antibacterial compounds that prevent cavities from forming.

Type 2 diabetes: Chocolate consumption was found to improve insulin response, most likely through the action of flavonoids.

HEALTH SPOTLIGHT

Reduced Risk of Heart Attack

Researchers at the Johns Hopkins University School of Medicine discovered a few squares of chocolate might be as beneficial to the heart as aspirin. They found that the blood platelets from study participants who ate chocolate took longer to clump together than those who had not (about 130 seconds compared to 123). The study concluded that eating a few squares a day may reduce heart attack risk by nearly 50 percent.

QUICK TIPS

❖ Look for dark chocolate with at least 70 percent cocoa content. Milk chocolate has *not* been found to have the same benefits as dark chocolate.

❖ Be sure to choose chocolate with no hydrogenated or partially hydrogenated oils.

Dark Chocolate

Truffles
YIELD: ABOUT 16 TRUFFLES

Matcha Truffles

4 ounces chocolate (70% or darker)
1 teaspoon matcha powder
Few drops toasted sesame oil
$^1/_2$ cup whipping cream
1 tablespoon agave nectar

Put the chocolate, matcha powder, and sesame oil in a small heat-safe bowl. In a small saucepan, heat the whipping cream and agave nectar. Simmer over low heat, stirring constantly for 1 minute. Pour the hot cream over the chocolate and whisk until smooth and glossy. Cool to room temperature. Cover and refrigerate overnight. When ready to assemble, follow instructions on page 93.

Rose-Cardamom Truffles

4 ounces chocolate (70% or darker)
$^1/_2$ teaspoon cardamom
$^1/_2$ cup whipping cream
$^1/_2$ ounce dried roses or lavender flowers
1 tablespoon agave nectar

Put the chocolate and cardamom in a small heat-safe bowl. In a small saucepan, over low heat, simmer the whipping cream, agave nectar, and dried flowers for 2 minutes. Pour the hot, infused cream through a sieve into the bowl of chocolate. Discard the flowers. Whisk the chocolate and cream until smooth and glossy. Cool to room temperature. Cover and refrigerate overnight. When ready to assemble, follow instructions on page 93.

Curry-Ginger Truffles

4 ounces chocolate (70% or darker)
$1/2$ ounce crystallized ginger, minced fine
$1/2$ cup whipping cream
1 tablespoon agave nectar
$1/2$ teaspoon sweet curry powder

In a heat-safe bowl, combine the chocolate and crystallized ginger. In a small saucepan, over low heat, simmer the whipping cream, agave nectar, and sweet curry powder for 1 minute. Pour the hot cream over the chocolate and ginger and whisk until smooth and glossy. Cool to room temperature. Cover and refrigerate overnight. When ready to assemble, follow instructions on page 93.

Mint-Lemon Truffles

4 ounces chocolate (70% or darker)
$1/2$ cup whipping cream
$1/2$ ounce fresh peppermint leaves
(about 50 large leaves)
1 teaspoon fresh grated lemon zest
1 tablespoon agave nectar

Put the chocolate in a small heat-safe bowl. In a small saucepan, over low heat, simmer the whipping cream, peppermint leaves, zest, and agave nectar for 2 minutes. Pour the infused hot cream through a sieve into the bowl of chocolate. Discard the mint leaves. Whisk the chocolate and cream until smooth and glossy. Cool to room temperature. Cover and refrigerate overnight. When ready to assemble, follow instructions on page 93.

Chipotle Truffles

4 ounces chocolate (70% or darker)
$1/2$ cup whipping cream
1 tablespoon agave nectar
$1/2$ vanilla bean, split and scraped
$1/4$ teaspoon chipotle powder
$1/2$ teaspoon pie spice

Put the chocolate in a small heat-safe bowl. In a small saucepan, over low heat, simmer the whipping cream, agave nectar, pod and seeds of the vanilla bean, chipotle powder, and pie spice for 2 minutes. Pour the hot cream through a sieve into the bowl of chocolate. Discard the vanilla bean pod. Whisk the chocolate until smooth and glossy. Cool to room temperature. Cover and refrigerate overnight. When ready to assemble, follow instructions below.

Chai-Coconut Truffles

4 ounces chocolate (70% or darker)
$1/2$ ounce finely minced, unsweetened dry coconut
$1/2$ cup whipping cream
1 tablespoon agave nectar
1 ounce loose chai tea

In a small heat-safe bowl, combine the chocolate and coconut. In a small saucepan, over low heat, simmer the whipping cream, agave nectar, and chai tea for 2 minutes. Pour the infused, hot cream through a sieve into the bowl of chocolate. Discard the tea. Whisk the chocolate and cream until smooth and glossy. Cool to room temperature. Cover and refrigerate overnight.

TO PREPARE TRUFFLES: Use a .5-ounce disher (like a small ice-cream scoop), available at restaurant supply stores. The disher ensures uniformity in size and makes rolling easier. But, if you don't have a disher, do not despair! You can get the job done with a teaspoon and a little elbow grease. For each truffle, portion out about a teaspoon (or one .5-ounce disher scoop) of the hardened mixture. Roll the portion between the palms of your hands until you have a small ball. This part can get messy, so work quickly with chilled mixture. Roll the mixture in unsweetened cocoa powder to coat. You can get creative and roll them in colored sprinkles or powdered sugar. The chai truffles can be rolled in finely minced unsweetened coconut. Keep truffles refrigerated until you are ready to serve them.

* * *

For other recipes and ways of using chocolate, see: Cranberry-Chocolate Tart (page 5), Chocolate-Chai Oatmeal (page 138), Chocolate-Peanut Butter Muesli (page 220).

21. DATES

Date palms grew in Egypt as early as the fifth century B.C. They were one of the few fruits able to grow in the hot climate of Egypt, and were common in the ancient Egyptian diet. In fact, Medjool dates (used in the recipe here) were once the most prized dates in the Mediterranean. It's easy to understand why. These dates are so sweet, they are often compared to candy. But although they are high in natural, unrefined sugars, they are rich in fiber, potassium, and B-complex vitamins. And phytochemicals present in fruit such as dates have been found to have antioxidant and anti-inflammatory effects that may be protective against health problems including cancer and heart disease.

HEALTH BENEFITS

Research shows compounds and nutrients found in dates may benefit:

Anemia: Iron is essential for oxygenation of blood and energy production; copper helps the body utilize iron.

Anxiety: B vitamins help reduce anxiety and have a calming effect on the nerves.

Breast cancer: Eating a diet high in fruit is associated with a lower risk of breast cancer.

Depression: B vitamins are necessary for the synthesis of the feel-good chemical serotonin that also helps regulate depression; low levels of B vitamins are linked to depression.

Fatigue: B vitamins, iron, and copper can boost low energy levels.

Healthy hair and skin color: Copper helps produce melanin, the pigment responsible for hair and skin color.

Heart health: Phytochemicals act as anti-inflammatories, protecting against inflammation associated with the onset of heart disease.

High blood pressure: Potassium lowers blood pressure.

High cholesterol: Fiber reduces cholesterol by binding bile and cholesterol together and helping to shuttle it out of the body.

Irritable bowel syndrome: Soluble fiber benefits symptoms including gas, pain, and bloating.

Migraine headache: Magnesium relaxes muscles and nerves and is often low in migraine sufferers.

Osteoporosis: Calcium is essential for building bone, while copper minimizes mineral loss that weakens bone.

PMS symptoms: Magnesium helps relieve symptoms including headache, bloating, and moodiness.

Stroke: Potassium lowers blood pressure and reduces the stickiness of blood platelets that can cause clotting.

Thyroid health: Copper is required for normal thyroid function (the gland that helps regulate body temperature and metabolism).

Wound healing: Studies show vitamin B5 can speed wound healing.

DATES NUTRITION INFORMATION

Serving Size 1 Medjool date, pitted	
Amount Per Serving	
Calories 66	Calories from fat 0
	% Daily Value
Total Fat 0 grams	0%
Saturated fat 0 gm	0%
Trans fat 0 gm	†
Cholesterol 0 milligrams	0%
Sodium 0 mg	0%
Total Carbohydrate 18 gm	6%
Dietary fiber 2 gm	8%
Sugars 16 gm	†
Protein 0 gm	0%
Vitamin A	1%
Vitamin C	0%
Calcium	2%
Iron	1%
Also contains:	
Potassium	5%
Copper	4%
Manganese	4%
Magnesium	3%
Vitamin B3 (niacin)	2%
Vitamin B5 (pantothenic acid)	2%
Vitamin B6 (pyridoxine)	2%

† Daily Value not established.
* Percent Daily Values are based on a 2,000-calorie diet.

HEALTH SPOTLIGHT

Dates Good for the Heart

Dates are rich in potassium, a mineral that's proving to be as important to keeping blood pressure at healthy levels as cutting salt intake. An analysis of 3,300 people involved in the Dallas Heart Study, a multi-ethnic investigation of cardiovascular disease, showed that those with the highest intakes of potassium in the diet had lower blood pressure. There was a significant association between study participants with high blood pressure and low-potassium diets. This remained true even after factors such as age, race, and other cardiovascular risk factors were considered.

QUICK TIPS

❖ Two tastes that taste great together: For a candy-bar taste that's loaded with nutrition, try spreading peanut butter on Medjool dates, or eat them with a handful of almonds.

❖ Dateland, Arizona, is famous for its date shakes, and it's a must-stop on a road trip through the state. Blend a handful of pitted dates into a vanilla milkshake to make your own date shake at home.

Stuffed Date Appetizer with Pomegranate Dipping Sauce

YIELD: 12 APPETIZERS

1 cup pomegranate 100% juice concentrate*

2 tablespoons sucanat

12 large Medjool dates

4 ounces chèvre (goat cheese)

1 4-ounce package prosciutto
(6 paper-thin slices)

Nonstick cooking spray

*A variety of pomegranate 100% juice concentrates are available in the frozen section of the supermarket. Our favorite brand is Old Orchard. For this recipe, use their pomegranate-cherry blend.

Preheat oven to 350°F.

In a small saucepan, over medium heat, combine juice concentrate and sucanat. Bring to a boil and stir to dissolve the sucanat. Turn heat down to very low. The mixture should not boil, but steam will rise off the surface. Cook over very low heat for 30 minutes. The mixture will have reduced slightly, by only about one-quarter. Allow the mixture to cool and set aside to use as a dipping sauce for dates when you are ready to serve.

Meanwhile, cut halfway through each date and remove the pit. Be careful not to cut completely through the date so that one side stays hinged. Stuff each date with approximately one-third of an ounce of chèvre. Cut each slice of prosciutto in half the long way so that you have 12 long, thin strips of prosciutto. Roll each stuffed date in a half slice of prociutto. Secure each roll with a toothpick.

Spray a baking sheet with nonstick cooking spray. Bake stuffed and wrapped dates on the baking sheet for 10 to 15 minutes, or just until the prosciutto starts to take on some color. Serve hot with the pomegranate dipping sauce.

* * *

For other recipes and ways of using dates, see: Date-Pine Nut Muesli (page 221).

22. FENNEL

Black licorice lovers, this is your vegetable. Fennel has a mild licorice flavor combined with a crunch similar to celery. The Romans used fennel as a digestive aid, and Roman women ate it in the belief it would help prevent obesity. The Greek physician Hippocrates prescribed fennel to increase breast milk in nursing women. It turns out fennel is loaded with antioxidants including the phytonutrient flavonoids rutin, kaempferol, and quercetin. In Italy, it is sometimes served as part of the dessert course, along with cheese and fruit. And it's often paired with seafood, including salmon. In this simple recipe, it's combined with mussels.

HEALTH BENEFITS

Research shows compounds and nutrients found in fennel may benefit:

Alzheimer's disease: Eating a diet high in folate was found to cut Alzheimer's risk by half.

Cancer (mouth, breast, ovarian, laryngeal, and esophageal cancers): Quercetin and anethole play a preventive role (see Health Spotlight).

Colon cancer: Research shows quercetin helps lower risk of pre-cancerous tumors.

Common cold: Quercetin plus vitamin C boost the immune system to fend off colds.

Depression: Kaempferol acts as an antidepressant.

Flu: Quercetin reduces the likelihood of getting the flu.

Heart attack: Folate, which lowered heart attack risk by 55 percent in one study, inhibits the formation of homocysteine (a potentially toxic chemical and significant risk factor for heart disease).

High blood pressure: Rutin may relax blood vessels; potassium lowers blood pressure.

High cholesterol: Fiber reduces cholesterol by binding bile and cholesterol together and helping to shuttle it out of the body.

Immunity: Vitamin C enhances the immune system's ability to fight ear infections, colds, and flu.

Irritable bowel syndrome: Soluble fiber relieves symptoms including gas, pain, and bloating.

Migraine headache: Magnesium relaxes muscles and nerves and is often low in migraine sufferers.

Osteo- and rheumatoid arthritis: Vitamin C reduces inflammation and free-radical damage within joints; it is also essential for production and maintenance of collagen, a major protein found in cartilage that helps cushion joints.

Osteoporosis: Calcium is essential for building and maintaining strong bones.

PMS symptoms: Manganese and magnesium help reduce symptoms, including headache, bloating, and moodiness.

FENNEL NUTRITION INFORMATION

Serving Size 1 medium fennel bulb

Amount Per Serving

Calories 73	Calories from fat 4

	% Daily Value
Total Fat 0 gm	0%
Saturated fat 0 gm	0%
Trans fat 0 gm	†
Cholesterol 0 milligrams	0%
Sodium 122 mg	5%
Total Carbohydrate 17 gm	6%
Dietary fiber 7 gm	29%
Sugars 0 gm	†
Protein 3 gm	6%
Vitamin A	6%
Vitamin C	47%
Calcium	11%
Iron	9%
Also contains:	
Potassium	28%
Manganese	22%
Folate	16%
Calcium	11%
Magnesium	10%
Copper	8%

† Daily Value not established.
* Percent Daily Values are based on a 2,000-calorie diet.

Pregnancy: Folate serves a critical function in growth and reproduction, and protects against a number of congenital malformations, including neural tube birth defects.

Type 2 diabetes: Rutin may decrease fasting blood sugar; low levels of manganese have been associated with diabetes.

HEALTH SPOTLIGHT

Fennel Fights Cancer

In addition to containing the cancer-fighter quercetin, fennel also has another cancer-fighting compound. A phytonutrient in fennel called anethole is a powerful anti-inflammatory that has been shown to help prevent cancer in several studies. It is believed that anethole works by shutting down signals in the cells that activate a molecule called NF-kappa B, responsible for inflammation and altered genes that can lead to cancer.

QUICK TIPS

❖ Add thinly sliced fennel to a baking pan with salmon, or wrap in foil along with salmon before baking.

❖ Add sliced fennel bulb to sandwiches along with lettuce and tomato, or drizzle with oil and vinegar for a simple salad.

❖ Don't throw fennel stalks and leaves away! The stalks are fantastic in soups and salads, and the leaves can be used as a seasoning—like the bulb, they have a licorice flavor.

Mussels in Fennel Broth

YIELD: 4 DINNER PORTIONS

3 pounds mussels, de-bearded and scrubbed

2 tablespoons olive oil

1 large brown onion, thinly sliced

2 medium fennel bulbs, fronds and core removed, thinly sliced

6 cloves garlic, crushed

$1/2$ teaspoon salt

1 bottle (8 ounces) clam juice

$1/2$ cup chardonnay (or other dry white wine)

$1/2$ teaspoon black pepper

1 tablespoon unsalted butter

4 servings linguini prepared according to package directions

Heat the olive oil in a large skillet. Add the onion, fennel, garlic, and salt. Sauté the mixture over low heat until the onions are translucent.

Add the clam juice, chardonnay, and pepper. Bring to a boil and simmer for 3 to 5 minutes until the sauce is reduced by about one-fourth its original volume. Reduce the heat to low. Pour the cleaned mussels into the broth. Cover with a tight-fitting lid. Cook over low heat 5 to 7 minutes, or until all the mussels are fully opened.

Remove from heat and immediately stir in the butter.

Divide the cooked pasta among four large bowls. Spoon the broth, mussels, and vegetables evenly among the bowls.

* * *

For other recipes and ways of using fennel, see: Roasted Beet and Fennel Salad (page 45), Salmon Quick Tips (page 178), Tomato-Seafood Chowder (203).

23. FIGS

"Figs are restorative, and the best food that can be taken
by those who are brought low by long sickness."
—PLINY, ROMAN NATURALIST (A.D. 23–79)

There is evidence that fig trees may have been the first-ever domesticated crop, dating as far back as 11,400 years. With ties to history, myth, and legend, the fig is endowed with an aura of mystique, and its unique combination of smooth, chewy, and crunchy textures makes it unlike any other fruit. Interestingly, figs contain a range of minerals that resembles that of breast milk, including phosphorus, iron, magnesium, manganese, calcium, and potassium. Additionally, they boast a high content of vitamin B_6 and folate, along with benzaldehyde, ficin, and mucin compounds. Fig leaves are also edible, and are surprisingly good for you.

HEALTH BENEFITS

Research shows compounds and nutrients found in figs and fig leaves may benefit:

Breast cancer: Fruit fiber is strongly associated with decreased risk in post-menopausal women.

Cancer: Polyphenols are protective against cancer; benzaldehyde has successfully treated cancer in studies.

Constipation: Ficin has laxative properties, as do fiber and magnesium; figs can be boiled to make a syrup and used as a laxative.

Diabetes: Fiber helps control blood sugar levels by slowing the release of glucose into the bloodstream; compounds in fig leaves may reduce the amount of insulin needed by diabetics (see Health Spotlight).

Digestive health: Ficin and enzymes help to break down protein, aiding in digestion.

Fatigue: Iron is essential for oxygenation of the blood and energy production; it relieves fatigue and along with fruit sugars boosts energy.

High blood pressure: Potassium lowers blood pressure.

High triglycerides: Fig leaves may lower harmful levels of triglycerides.

Immunity: Vitamin B_6 aids in immune system function and in antibody production.

Macular degeneration (age-related): Eating three or more servings of fruit a day is linked to decreased risk.

PMS symptoms: Manganese helps relieve cramping and mood swings.

Osteoporosis: Calcium is essential for building and maintaining strong bones.

Sexual health: Folate may boost sperm production; figs are also said to be an aphrodisiac.

Weight loss and weight control: Fiber-containing foods provide a

feeling of fullness; fiber slows digestion, helping to keep blood sugar levels stable and reduce insulin spikes that can trigger cravings and encourage fat storage.

FIGS NUTRITION INFORMATION

Serving Size 1 large fig, raw

Amount Per Serving

Calories 47	Calories from fat 2
	% Daily Value
Total Fat 0 grams	0%
Saturated fat 0 gm	0%
Trans fat 0 gm	†
Cholesterol 0 milligrams	0%
Sodium 1 mg	.04%
Total Carbohydrate 12 gm	4%
Dietary fiber 2 gm	7%
Sugars 10 gm	†
Protein 0 gm	0%
Vitamin A	2%
Vitamin C	2%
Calcium	2%
Iron	1%
Also contains:	
Potassium	4%
Manganese	4%
Vitamin B_6 (pyridoxine)	4%
Vitamin K	4%
Magnesium	3%

† Daily Value not established.
* Percent Daily Values are based on a 2,000-calorie diet.

QUICK TIP

❖ For an amazing appetizer, wrap prosciutto slices around fresh fig halves or quarters. Hold in place with toothpicks and arrange on a serving platter.

HEALTH SPOTLIGHT

Fig Leaves Beneficial in Diabetes

Research shows that fig leaves have anti-diabetic properties. In one study, a liquid extract made from fig leaves was added to the breakfasts of insulin-dependent diabetic subjects. Results showed the extract reduced the amount of insulin needed by the test subjects. Fig leaves are difficult to come by in stores, but if you have a fig tree, you can incorporate the leaves into your diet by wrapping them around fish or meat before baking or grilling. Or simply boil the leaves to make a "tea." They have been used in cooking for centuries by the Greeks and Romans.

Roasted Fig and Cheese Appetizer

YIELD: 32 TO 36 APPETIZERS

8 to 9 ounces (8 to 9 large) fresh figs

2 tablespoons olive oil

$1/4$ cup balsamic vinegar

$1/4$ cup honey

4 ounces chèvre (goat) cheese log or mini-round brie

32 to 36 whole-grain crackers

Preheat oven to 350°F.

Trim the stems from the figs and quarter them. Put the figs into a 9-by-9-inch baking pan. In a small bowl, whisk the olive oil, vinegar, and the honey until well blended. Pour the mixture over the figs and toss to coat. Roast for 40 minutes, tossing to coat the figs with syrup every 10 minutes. Place the cheese log or round on a serving platter and allow it to come to room temperature. Pour the hot figs and their syrup over the cheese and serve with crackers.

24. GOJI BERRIES

Nicknamed the "happy berry," goji berries are said to make you happy all day when you eat them in the morning. In fact, folk medicine purports that the berries cause you to laugh more than usual. Also known as wolfberry, tiny red goji berries are loaded with vitamins A and C, along with other antioxidants and compounds including betaine, physalin, and polysaccharides, that have been shown to benefit a wide range of conditions. These studies seem to back up claims that goji berries are one of the reasons the people of the Himalayas, where they have grown for more than 3,000 years, live long and healthy lives, and lend support to the wisdom of Chinese herbalists, who have been prescribing them for centuries to increase sexual potency. For some, their taste is an acquired one, but even if you're not crazy about the taste of goji berries, you'll love them in this recipe.

HEALTH BENEFITS

Research shows compounds and nutrients found in goji berries may benefit:

Allergies: Goji berries appear to reduce antibodies associated with allergic reactions.

Alzheimer's disease: Goji berries appear to have neuroprotective effects.

Anxiety: Goji berry juice drinkers reported feeling less stressed after two weeks.

Cancer: In a study, cancer patients responded better to treatment when goji berries were added to their treatment regimens; test-tube research also demonstrates an anti-cancer effect.

Concentration: Betaine is converted into choline, a substance that helps enhance memory and recall ability.

Depression: Goji berry juice increases feelings of happiness and well-being.

Diabetes: Goji berries may improve insulin resistance.

Eyesight: Goji berries' high antioxidant content may benefit night blindness, and blurred and poor vision.

Fatigue: People who drank goji berry juice for fourteen days reported increased energy.

Fertility in men: Polysaccharides protect DNA in testicle cells.

Healthy skin and nails: In one study, the health of skin and nails improved with drinking goji berry juice.

Heart health: Antioxidants help prevent dangerous levels of homocysteine from accumulating.

Immunity: Goji berries show promise in immunity, possibly due to their vitamin C content and other compounds including polysaccharides.

GOJI BERRIES NUTRITION INFORMATION	
Serving Size 40 grams (a small handful) of goji berries	
Amount Per Serving	
Calories 150	Calories from fat 0
	% Daily Value*
Total Fat 0 grams	0%
Saturated fat 0 gm	0%
Trans fat 0 gm	†
Cholesterol 0 milligrams	0%
Sodium 190 mg	8%
Total Carbohydrate 32 gm	11%
Dietary fiber 1 gm	5%
Sugars 30 gm	†
Protein 5 gm	10%
Vitamin A	20%
Vitamin C	10%
Calcium	0%
Iron	8%
† Daily Value not established.	
* Percent Daily Values are based on a 2,000-calorie diet.	

Leukemia: Physalin may inhibit the growth of leukemia cells.

Liver protection: Betaine may work to protect the liver.

Longevity: Antioxidants help protect against the formation of free radicals, which promote aging and disease.

Menstrual cramps: Women who drank goji berry juice for two weeks experienced a decrease in cramps.

Osteo- and rheumatoid arthritis: Goji berries contain anti-inflammatory polysaccharides that help reduce arthritis-related pain.

Sleep quality: Goji berry juice appears to help promote a good night's sleep.

HEALTH SPOTLIGHT

Goji Berry Juice Makes You Happy

One study showed a variety of positive effects from drinking goji berry juice, including "contentment and happiness." Thirty-five people were given either goji berry juice or a placebo every morning for two weeks. After the test period, 50 to 60 percent of the goji berry juice drinkers reported feeling "good health, contentment and happiness." Other reported benefits from this same study included a decrease in menstrual cramps, an increase in sexual activity, and healthier skin and nails!

QUICK TIPS

❖ Steep dried goji berries in a cup of hot tea along with the tea leaves. They add flavor and nutrients to the tea, and the tea also "plumps up" and mellows the flavor of the berries.

❖ Try goji berries with hot or cold cereal in the morning.

Goji Berry Granola

YIELD: APPROXIMATELY 5 CUPS

2 cups rolled oats

$1^1/_2$ cups chopped walnuts

$1/_2$ cup wheat bran

$1^1/_2$ cups goji berries

2 tablespoons matcha powder

1 teaspoon ground cardamom

$1/_2$ cup agave nectar

$1/_4$ cup sucanat

2 tablespoons safflower, peanut, grape seed, or walnut oil

1 tablespoon vanilla extract

$1/_2$ teaspoon salt

Nonstick cooking spray

Preheat oven to 200°F.

In a large bowl, combine the oats, walnuts, wheat bran, goji berries, matcha powder, and cardamom. Mix well and set aside for later use.

In a small saucepan, combine well the agave nectar, sucanat, oil, vanilla, and salt. Cook over low heat just until the sucanat is completely dissolved and forms a syrup. Pour into the oat mixture. Stir well so that all the oats and fruit are completely covered in the syrup.

Spray a 12-by-17-inch baking sheet with nonstick cooking spray. Evenly spread the granola on the baking sheet. Bake for 2 hours and 10 minutes. Use a spatula to turn the granola approximately every half hour. Allow the granola to cool completely in the pan on a cooling rack. Break apart into bite-size chunks. Store the granola in an airtight container.

*   *   *

For other recipes and ways of using goji berries, see: Goji-Cardamom Muesli (page 221).

25. GRAPEFRUIT

The grapefruit, with its unique tart-bitter-sweet taste, is thought to be the result of a natural cross-pollination of a pomelo and an orange. It was first discovered in Barbados in the 1700s and dubbed the "forbidden fruit" by religious scholars of the time who believed it was the "apple" mentioned in the Bible. But you should welcome this fruit in your diet. The grapefruit offers a one-of-a-kind array of nutrients including not only high doses of both vitamins A and C, but also of lycopene and limonoids (both of which have been shown to fight cancer), and powerful citrus flavonoids including naringin, naringenin, and tangeretin.

HEALTH BENEFITS

Research shows compounds and nutrients found in grapefruit may benefit:

Alzheimer's disease: Grapefruit juice may slow progression of the disease by reducing the accumulation of brain-damaging plaque.

Asthma: Vitamin C reduces inflammation that can restrict airways.

Breast cancer: Liminoids may prevent breast cancer cells from proliferating by promoting the formation of glutathione, a powerful antioxidant that helps break down toxins and carcinogens.

Cataracts: Diets high in citrus fruits are associated with lower risk.

Colon cancer: Liminoids may prevent colon cancer cells from proliferating (see Breast cancer).

Common cold: Vitamin C boosts immunity and may reduce cold symptoms.

Detox: Compounds in grapefruit boost enzymes in the liver that help clear out toxins and carcinogens.

Diabetes: Grapefruit may reduce the amount of insulin required to lower blood sugar after a meal.

Gingivitis: Vitamin C promotes healing, especially of bleeding gums.

Heart health: Lycopene is associated with reduced risk of cardiovascular disease.

High cholesterol: Grapefruit pectin may help dissolve arterial plaque that results from a high-cholesterol diet.

Kidney stones: Daily consumption of grapefruit juice may help promote citric acid excretion, significantly reducing risk of stone formation.

Longevity: Antioxidants help protect against the formation of free radicals, which promote aging and disease.

Lung cancer: A 6-ounce glass of grapefruit juice a day may help protect against cancer-causing chemicals in tobacco smoke.

GRAPEFRUIT NUTRITION INFORMATION

Serving Size 1/2 grapefruit

Amount Per Serving

Calories 52		Calories from fat 1
		% Daily Value*
Total Fat 0 grams		0%
Saturated fat 0 gm		0%
Trans fat 0 gm		†
Cholesterol 0 milligrams		0%
Sodium 0 mg		0%
Total Carbohydrate 13 gm		4%
Dietary fiber 2 gm		8%
Sugars 8 gm		†
Protein 1 gm		2%
Vitamin A		28%
Vitamin C		64%
Calcium		3%
Iron		1%

† Daily Value not established.
* Percent Daily Values are based on a 2,000-calorie diet.

Macular degeneration (age-related): Eating three or more servings of fruit a day is linked to decreased risk.

Osteo- and rheumatoid arthritis: Vitamin C reduces inflammation and free-radical damage within joints; it is also essential for production and maintenance of collagen, a major protein found in cartilage that helps cushion joints.

Parkinson's disease: Tangeretin increased dopamine levels in one study and may have neuroprotective effects.

Prostate cancer: Naringenin shows promise in promoting the repair of damaged DNA in prostate cells.

Skin health: Vitamin C aids in collagen formation and protects against free-radical damage.

Stroke: Vitamin C intake is associated with lower risk of stroke.

Weight control and weight loss: Grapefruit may aid weight loss by lowering insulin levels.

HEALTH SPOTLIGHT

Super Prostate Cancer Fighter

A study published in the *Journal of Nutritional Biochemistry* reports that a flavonoid in grapefruit called naringenin can repair damaged DNA in the prostate. In the study, scientists exposed cell cultures to naringenin and found that the flavonoid activated two DNA-repairing enzymes. Grapefruit also contains lycopene, another prostate-cancer fighter. Note: In another study, grapefruit was associated with an increased risk of breast cancer in post-menopausal women. Grapefruit can also interfere with some medications. Check with your doctor.

QUICK TIP

❖ Here's a great way to start the day: sprinkle some cinnamon on half a grapefruit.

Grapefruit Breakfast Napoleon

YIELD: 2 NAPOLEONS

3 tablespoons sucanat or light brown sugar

$3/4$ teaspoon ground cardamom

2 8-inch multigrain tortillas, cut into quarters

2 to 3 tablespoons safflower oil

6 ounces Greek-style yogurt

2 8-ounce pink grapefruits, supremed
(see directions on page 47)

2 ounces salted pistachios, toasted and coarsely chopped
(see directions on following page)

Toasting Nuts

To toast pistachios (or any other nut), preheat oven to 350°F. Place the nuts in a single layer on an ungreased baking sheet. Bake for 5 to 10 minutes or until they are golden brown. Turn once with a spatula during cooking so that they brown evenly. Watch them closely, being careful not to burn them. Remove from pan to cool.

Preheat oven to 350°F.

In a small dish, combine the sucanat and the cardamom. Place tortilla quarters on a baking sheet and lightly brush with oil. Sprinkle about two-thirds of the sugar mixture on the tortilla quarters. Bake for 8 to 10 minutes, until tortillas are crisp and sucanat just begins to bubble. Remove tortillas to a cooling rack and set aside for later use.

While the tortilla quarters are baking, supreme the grapefruits and roast the nuts.

Turn the oven up to the broil setting. On a clean baking sheet, lay grapefruit segments out so that they are not touching. Sprinkle the remaining sucanat mixture over the grapefruit segments. Broil the grapefruit segments for 3 minutes.

TO ASSEMBLE THE NAPOLEONS: Stack the recipe elements in this order: tortilla, dollop of yogurt, approximately one-sixth of the grapefruit segments, a sprinkling of pistachios. Repeat this pattern until you have three layers and finish with a tortilla quarter on top. You have enough to make 2 complete stacks.

26. MANGOES

This exotic tropical fruit has been cultivated for at least 4,000 years, with origins in Asia and India. Today, the mango is one of the most popular fresh fruits in the world. Mangoes feature an amazing combination of antioxidant phenolic compounds including gallic acid (also present in dark chocolate), coumaric acid (shown to inhibit the development of stomach cancer), tannic acid (shown to have antibacterial properties), and protocatechuic acid (shown to inhibit tumor growth). Mangoes also contain the antioxidants quercetin and norathyriol (a compound that may help regulate glucose), an abundance of antioxidants like vitamins A and C, and omega-3 fatty acids.

HEALTH BENEFITS

Research shows compounds and nutrients found in mangoes may benefit:

Allergies: Gallic acid suppresses the release of histamines (chemicals that cause allergic reactions), which decreases allergy symptoms like itchy, watery eyes and sneezing.

Alzheimer's disease: Gallic acid shows promise in protecting brain cells; omega-3s may slow progression of the disease by reducing the accumulation of brain-damaging plaque.

Anxiety: Vitamin B_6 helps reduce anxiety and exerts a calming effect.

Asthma: Phenols and vitamin C have anti-inflammatory effects in lungs.

Cancer (colon and lung cancers, and leukemia): Gallic acid and protocatechuic acid may be cancer protective.

Depression: Vitamin B_6 is necessary for the synthesis of the feel-good chemical serotonin that helps lift mood and fight depression.

Flu: Quercetin reduces the likelihood of getting the flu.

Heart attack and stroke: Quercetin reduces plaque buildup.

Immunity: Vitamins A and C are powerful antioxidants that decrease susceptibility to infection.

Irritable bowel syndrome: Soluble fiber benefits symptoms including gas, pain, and bloating.

Macular degeneration (age-related): Vitamins A and C are associated with a reduced risk of age-related macular degeneration.

Night blindness: Vitamin A improves nighttime vision by increasing retinol (the most usable form of vitamin A).

Osteo- and rheumatoid arthritis: Antioxidants (especially vitamin C) and anti-inflammatories limit free-radical damage and inflammation and reduce arthritis-related pain.

Prostate cancer: Quercetin may inhibit hormone activity in prostate cancer cell lines.

Skin health: Vitamin C aids in collagen formation and protects against free-radical damage.

MANGOES NUTRITION INFORMATION

Serving Size 1 cup mango, sliced

Amount Per Serving

Calories 107		Calories from fat 4
		% Daily Value*
Total Fat 0 grams		0%
Saturated fat 0 gm		0%
Trans fat 0 gm		†
Cholesterol 0 milligrams		0%
Sodium 0 mg		0%
Total Carbohydrate 28 gm		9%
Dietary fiber 3 gm		12%
Sugars 24 gm		†
Protein 1 gm		2%
Vitamin A		25%
Vitamin C		76%
Calcium		2%
Iron		1%
Also contains:		
Omega-3 fatty acids 61.1 mg		†
Vitamin B$_6$ (pyridoxine)		11%
Vitamin E		9%

† Daily Value not established.
* Percent Daily Values are based on a 2,000-calorie diet.

Stomach cancer: Coumaric acid may inhibit the development of stomach cancer.

Type 2 diabetes: Norathyriol may protect against diabetes by encouraging the efficient use of glucose.

HEALTH SPOTLIGHT

Mangoes for Allergies

Mangoes contain gallic acid, a polyphenyl also found in green tea that has anti-inflammatory properties, in addition to antioxidant and antimicrobial activity. In a study, gallic acid was shown to block histamine release, and could have therapeutic use in decreasing allergy symptoms like itchy, watery eyes and sneezing. Another compound in mangoes, quercetin, has also been shown to prevent histamine release.

QUICK TIPS

❖ Sprinkle mango with salt or dip into soy sauce as they do in the Philippines.

❖ For yummy appetizers, serve crackers with cream cheese and mango chutney.

❖ Try dried mango with cayenne pepper.

Mango and Herb Pasta with Peanut Sauce

YIELD: 4 SERVINGS

Chicken

$1^1/_2$ cups coconut milk

$^1/_4$ cup lime juice

1 tablespoon sweet curry powder*

$^1/_2$ teaspoon salt

12 chicken breast tenders (about $1^1/_4$ pounds)

Sauce

$^1/_4$ cup toasted sesame oil

$^1/_3$ cup minced shallots

4 cloves garlic, minced

1 tablespoon minced ginger

1 tablespoon sweet curry powder*

*Our favorite is Penzeys Sweet Curry Powder.

$^1/_2$ cup coconut milk

2 tablespoons honey

$^1/_2$ cup fresh squeezed lime juice

Zest from squeezed limes (zest before juicing)

$^1/_2$ teaspoon kosher salt

$^1/_2$ cup natural, no sugar added, chunky peanut butter

Pasta

3 cups diced mango

2 scallions, green and white parts, thinly sliced

2 tablespoons minced fresh basil leaves

1 tablespoon minced fresh mint leaves

$^1/_4$ cup minced cilantro

4 ounces buckwheat pasta

2 tablespoons safflower, peanut, or grape seed oil

TO PREPARE THE CHICKEN: In a casserole dish or medium bowl, whisk the coconut milk, lime juice, curry powder, and salt together. Add the chicken tenders. Toss to coat. Refrigerate at least 2 hours.

TO PREPARE THE SAUCE: In a medium saucepan, over low heat, warm the sesame oil. Add the shallots, garlic, and ginger. Stir over low heat about 2 minutes, until soft and fragrant. Stir in the curry powder and continue to cook about 1 minute longer. Stir in the coconut milk, honey, lime juice, zest, and salt. Bring up to a simmer and whisk in the peanut butter. The sauce can be made ahead and reheated before serving.

Combine the mango, scallions, basil, mint, and cilantro in a large bowl and set aside for later use. Cook the pasta according to the package directions. Meanwhile, remove the tenders from the marinade and discard the marinade. Heat the oil in a large skillet. Cook the tenders over high heat, turning once to brown on both sides. Tenders will take 2 to 3 minutes per side to cook. Drain the pasta and while hot add it to the bowl with the herbs and mango. Toss well to combine. Divide the pasta among four plates. Drizzle the sauce over the pasta. Top each plate with three chicken tenders and serve immediately.

* * *

For other recipes and ways of using mango, see: Avocado Quick Tips (page 37).

27. MAPLE SYRUP

This nutrient-rich syrup is sweeter than sugar and a healthier alternative to sugar. Rather than providing only empty calories, maple syrup is rich in minerals including zinc (also an antioxidant), potassium, calcium, magnesium, and manganese. (Maple syrup contains a whopping 531 percent of the Daily Value of manganese per cup!) This natural sweetener is not only great poured on pancakes, but can be substituted for sugar in baking, or used to sweeten coffee or tea. Make sure to purchase only pure maple syrup (made by reducing the sap from maple trees)—not maple-flavored syrups with added artificial ingredients. Real, Grade-A maple syrup comes in light, medium, and dark amber versions according to a U.S. Department of Agriculture rating (the darker the syrup, the richer the flavor). Use your favorite in the maple muffins here, which make a great grab-and-go breakfast, or sweet addition to a sit-down Sunday brunch.

HEALTH BENEFITS

Research shows compounds and nutrients found in maple syrup may benefit:

Acne: Zinc may help prevent acne and regulate the activity of oil glands, and is often low in acne sufferers.

Alzheimer's disease: Zinc supplementation has been shown to improve memory, communication, and social contact.

Bone health: Manganese is vital for bone formation; a deficiency can cause abnormal skeletal development and bone loss (see Health Spotlight).

Brain function: Teens who took zinc performed better on memory tests than a control group.

Cell protection: Manganese activates the antioxidant enzyme superoxide dismutase (SOD), which protects the mitochondria (the energy-producing part of cells) from free-radical damage.

Common cold: Zinc lozenges are reported to reduce the severity and duration of cold symptoms.

Depression: Zinc deficiency is associated with depression; zinc may activate the production of brain-derived neurotropic factor, a substance needed to ward off depression.

Eye health: Zinc is a component of key enzymes that help preserve vision and protect against age-related vision loss; low levels in eye tissues may correlate with age-related macular degeneration.

Fertility in men: Zinc increases sperm production and male fertility.

Heart health: Potassium lowers blood pressure; magnesium dilates the coronary arteries, which improves blood flow to the heart, prevents blood platelets from clumping, and stabilizes heart rhythm.

Immunity: Zinc promotes immune-cell activity; even a mild deficiency can impair immune function and increase susceptibility to infections.

Metabolism: Manganese activates necessary enzymes responsible for healthy metabolism.

MAPLE SYRUP NUTRITION INFORMATION	
Serving Size 1 cup maple syrup	
Amount Per Serving	
Calories 840	Calories from fat 5
	% Daily Value*
Total Fat 1 gram	1%
Saturated fat 0 gm	0%
Trans fat 0 gm	†
Cholesterol 0 milligrams	0%
Sodium 29 mg	1%
Total Carbohydrate 216 gm	72%
Dietary fiber 0 gm	0%
Sugars 192 gm	†
Protein 0 gm	0%
Vitamin A	0%
Vitamin C	0%
Calcium	22%
Iron	21%
Also contains:	
Manganese	531%
Zinc	89%
Potassium	19%
Copper	12%
Magnesium	11%
† Daily Value not established.	
* Percent Daily Values are based on a 2,000-calorie diet.	

Rheumatoid arthritis: Zinc fights inflammation and may protect cartilage.

Thyroid health: Zinc may improve hypothyroidism, a condition marked by abnormally low thyroid hormone that can lead to weight gain.

Tinnitus: Zinc is concentrated in the inner ear and can help alleviate ringing in the ears.

Type 2 diabetes: Zinc may reduce risk for diabetes by helping regulate insulin function.

Wound healing: Manganese activates an enzyme called prolidase that is responsible for forming collagen.

HEALTH SPOTLIGHT

Postmenopausal Osteoporosis

One study, involving healthy postmenopausal women monitored over the course of two years, showed that manganese supplementation combined with zinc, copper, and calcium supplements—all nutrients found in maple syrup—reduced spinal bone loss more than a calcium supplement alone.

QUICK TIPS

❖ You can substitute pure maple syrup in recipes that call for sugar—use $3/4$ cup of pure maple syrup in place of each cup of sugar, and reduce the liquids in the recipe by three tablespoons.

❖ Your kids will love this, and you'll feel like a kid again—pour maple syrup over shaved ice for maple syrup snow cones.

Whole-Wheat Maple Schmootz Muffins

YIELD: 12 MUFFINS

Muffin Batter
$1/4$ cup butter
$1/2$ cup pure maple syrup
2 large eggs
1 cup buttermilk
$1/2$ teaspoon salt

1 teaspoon cinnamon

1 teaspoon vanilla extract

$1/2$ teaspoon baking powder

$1/2$ cup whole-wheat flour

$1/4$ cup flax meal

1 cup rolled oats

$1/4$ cup almond meal

$1/2$ cup wheat bran

2 tablespoons rice bran

Schmootz

$1/4$ cup unsalted butter

$1/2$ cup pure maple syrup

Preheat oven to 350°F.

TO MAKE THE BATTER: In the bowl of a stand mixer, beat the butter on low to soften. Add the maple syrup slowly to combine well. Add the eggs and buttermilk. With the mixer on low speed, add the remaining batter ingredients. Scrape down the sides of the bowl as necessary. Allow the batter to rest while you make the schmootz.

TO MAKE THE SCHMOOTZ: In the bowl of a food processor, fitted with the chopping blade, soften the butter. Slowly add the maple syrup to create a very liquid compound butter. The mixture may look curdled—that's okay. Scrape down the sides and process until the butter is evenly distributed throughout the maple syrup. Divide the schmootz evenly among 12 muffin cups (about 1 tablespoon per cup). Do not use paper muffin liners.

Next, divide the batter evenly among the 12 muffin cups. Just plop the batter right on top of the schmootz. Bake for 30 minutes. Remove from the oven. Immediately invert the muffin pan on a baking sheet. Muffins should fall out and be schmootz-covered.

* * *

For other recipes and ways of using maple syrup, see: Pumpkin Pots de Soymilk (page 165), Smoky Sweet Potatoes (page 200), Apple-Cinnamon Muesli (page 221).

28. MATCHA

"Tea is the ultimate mental and medical remedy and has the ability to make one's life more full and complete."

BUDDHIST PRIEST MYOAN ESAI,
TWELFTH CENTURY

Matcha is a green tea powder first cultivated during the Song Dynasty (960–1279) in China. It provides all the benefits of brewed green tea, only many times more concentrated. Because it is made from entire green tea leaves, which are ground into a fine talcum-like powder, all the nutrients and flavonoids remain—nothing is lost in brewing. Buddhist monks have sipped it for centuries—perhaps its L-theanine content, an amino acid said to promote relaxation and slow brain waves (despite its caffeine content), helped them achieve a state of zen. It is also widely cultivated in Japan and is a central part of traditional Japanese tea ceremonies. In China, green tea beverages including matcha have been used medicinally for millennia. Science is now revealing the compounds in green tea that make it so good for you, including catechins, epigallocatechin-3-gallate (EGCG), and polyphenols. Take a look.

HEALTH BENEFITS

Research shows compounds found in matcha may benefit:

Alzheimer's disease and Parkinson's disease: Catechins help destroy free radicals and protect against brain-cell death; EGCG has been shown to remove excess iron from the brain associated with these diseases.

Atherosclerosis: Green tea improves the flexibility of blood vessels and makes them less susceptible to clogging and hardening of the arteries.

Bladder cancer: Green tea is associated with a reduced risk of bladder cancer as well as a higher survival rate.

Blood clots: Catechins prevent the formation of pro-inflammatory compounds that cause platelets to stick together.

Brain health: Drinking green tea was associated with lower incidence of cognitive impairment in one study; tannins may help prevent brain damage.

Breast cancer: Increased green tea consumption before and after surgery reduced tumor growth and recurrence.

MATCHA NUTRITION INFORMATION		
Serving Size 1/2 teaspoon matcha		
Amount Per Serving		
Calories 3	Calories from fat 0	
		% Daily Value*
Total Fat 0 grams		0%
Sodium 0 milligrams		0%
Total Carbohydrate 0 gm		0%
Dietary fiber 0 gm		0%
Protein 0 gm		0%
* Percent Daily Values are based on a 2,000-calorie diet.		

Coronary heart disease: Polyphenols guard against free-radical damage to blood vessels that can lead to coronary artery disease.

Depression: Polyphenols can boost dopamine production in the brain, linked to mood.

Exercise endurance: Catechins encourage your body to burn fatty acids stored in muscles; regular consumption increases exercise endurance.

Flu: EGCG significantly slows replication of the flu virus.

Gallstones: Drinking one cup of green tea a day shows promise in reducing gallstone risk.

Gingivitis: Catechins inhibit effects of bacteria responsible for gum disease.

High blood pressure: Drinking two-and-a-half cups of green tea per day could lower high blood pressure risk by up to 65 percent.

High triglycerides: Catechins slow triglyceride production after meals.

Liver health: Polyphenols protect the liver from alcohol and carcinogens.

Longevity: Drinking green tea lowers risk of death due to all causes, including cancer and cardiovascular disease (see Health Spotlight).

Lung cancer: Catechins, especially EGCG, may work to inhibit cancer cell growth.

Osteoporosis: EGCG increases bone density.

Ovarian cancer: Polyphenols and catechins, especially EGCG, are cancer protective.

Prostate cancer: Catechins inhibit prostate specific antigen (PSA) production, an indicator of prostate cancer risk.

Rheumatoid arthritis: Green tea works to prevent overproduction of inflammatory cyclooxygenase-2 (COX-2), much like prescription drugs.

Stress management: L-theanine promotes relaxation by stimulating alpha brain waves, regarded as the healthiest brain-wave range.

Stroke: Catechins stop free radicals from developing in brain tissue, protecting the brain against damage due to stroke and heart attack.

Type 2 diabetes: EGCG helps regulate glucose levels by increasing insulin sensitivity.

Weight loss: Research shows green tea drinkers lost more body fat while on a calorie-controlled diet than a control group.

HEALTH SPOTLIGHT

Increase Longevity with Green Tea

A 2006 study published in the *Journal of the American Medical Association* found that drinking green tea lowers risk of death due to *all* causes, including cancer and cardiovascular disease. The study tracked 40,530 people in Japan, ages forty to seventy-nine, over the course of eleven years. About 80 percent of the study subjects drank green tea. More than half of these drank at least three cups a day. When compared to study subjects who drank less than one cup a day, researchers found a significantly lower risk of death from all causes, especially in women. Among those who drank five cups of green tea a day, women had a 23 percent lower risk, and men had a 12 percent lower risk of dying from any cause.

QUICK TIPS

❖ Make your own green tea ice cream: Mix matcha with vanilla ice cream.

❖ Add a scoop of matcha to your water bottle and sip throughout the day or after a workout.

❖ Whip up a green tea soy latte at home: Mix about 2 teaspoons of matcha with a cup of soymilk (sweetened or plain, depending on your taste). Heat on low and whisk until matcha is dissolved; add a dash of ginger if desired.

Matcha Panna Cotta

YIELD: 8 SERVINGS

2 teaspoons or one $1/4$-ounce envelope of gelatin

2 cups whipping cream

2 cups Greek-style yogurt

2 tablespoons matcha powder

1 vanilla bean, split lengthwise

$1/2$ cup unrefined cane sugar or sucanat

Nonstick cooking spray

1 pint berries for serving

In a small bowl, bloom the gelatin in $1/4$ cup of the whipping cream. Set aside for later use.

In a large bowl, combine the yogurt and matcha powder. Set aside for later use.

In a 1-quart saucepan, combine the remaining whipping cream and sucanat. Scrape the seeds from the vanilla bean and add the seeds and the pod to the cream. Bring the mixture to a simmer over low heat and dissolve the sucanat. Remove from heat. Stir in the bloomed gelatin until completely dissolved. Remove and discard the vanilla bean.

Whisking constantly, pour the vanilla cream into the yogurt/matcha mixture in a thin stream. Spray eight small custard cups with nonstick cooking spray. Divide the matcha mixture evenly among the custard cups and refrigerate overnight. To serve, invert the custard cup on a dessert plate and top with the berries.

*   *   *

For other recipes and ways of using matcha, see: Matcha Truffles (page 91), Goji Berry Granola (page 107), Matcha-Blueberry Muesli (page 221).

29. MILLET

No, not the bad haircut. Millet is actually a whole grain, and when it comes to grains it is one of the healthiest. Millet is gluten-free, versatile, and delicious. Depending on how you cook millet, it can have a creamy consistency or a fluffy consistency similar to rice. Whole grains like millet contain phytonutrient phenolics and lignans that work to lower cancer risk, along with polyunsaturated fatty acids such as omega-3 fatty acids, oligosaccharides, plant sterols, stanols, and saponins that help to lower cholesterol. And like fruits and vegetables, millet is abundant in antioxidant disease-fighters including selenium, phenolic acids, and phytic acid.

HEALTH BENEFITS

Research shows compounds and nutrients found in millet may benefit:

Asthma: Eating a diet that includes plenty of whole grains was found to cut risk of childhood asthma by 50 percent and reduce symptoms such as wheezing; magnesium may have a bronchodilating effect.

Bone health: Phosphorus works with calcium to keep bones strong.

Breast cancer: Lignans that are converted to enterolactone are thought to protect against hormone-related cancers; the higher the consumption of whole grains, the higher the level of this protective lignan.

Colon cancer: Eating a diet high in whole grains was found to lower risk of colon cancer, possibly because insoluble fiber moves harmful toxins and cancer-causing substances out of the colon more quickly.

Depression: Niacin aids in the functioning of the nervous system; vitamin B_6 helps synthesize the feel-good chemical serotonin that helps lift mood and fight depression.

Energy: Phosphorus is essential to production of adenosine triphosphate (ATP), the molecule that helps store energy in the body.

Gallstones: One large-scale study found that a high-fiber diet could reduce risk of gallstones by 17 percent (see Health Spotlight).

Heart attack risk: Magnesium improves blood flow to the heart, prevents blood platelets from clumping together, and stabilizes heart rhythm; magnesium deficiency may increase risk of heart attack.

Heart disease: In women, six servings of whole grains a week helped slow progression of atherosclerosis.

Heart failure: Eating whole-grain cereal for breakfast was found to lower heart failure risk by 29 percent.

High blood pressure: Magnesium promotes normal blood pressure.

High cholesterol: Polyunsaturated fatty acids, oligosaccharides, plant sterols and stanols, and saponins have been shown to lower cholesterol, possibly by keeping it from being absorbed into the bloodstream.

Insomnia: Millet contains tryptophan, a precursor for the neurotransmitter serotonin, which helps to regulate sleep.

MILLET NUTRITION INFORMATION	
Serving Size 1 cup millet, cooked	
Amount Per Serving	
Calories 207	Calories from fat 15
	% Daily Value*
Total Fat 2 grams	3%
Saturated fat 0 gm	0%
Trans fat 0 gm	†
Cholesterol 0 milligrams	0%
Sodium 3 mg	.125%
Total Carbohydrate 41 gm	14%
Dietary fiber 2 gm	9%
Sugars 0 gm	†
Protein 6 gm	12%
Vitamin A	0%
Vitamin C	0%
Calcium	1%
Iron	6%
Also contains:	
Manganese	24%
Magnesium	19%
Phosphorus	17%
Copper	14%
Vitamin B_1 (thiamine)	12%
Vitamin B_3 (niacin)	12%
Vitamin B_6 (pyridoxine)	9%
Folate	8%
Selenium	2%
Omega-3 fatty acids 48.7 mg	†
† Daily Value not established.	
* Percent Daily Values are based on a 2,000-calorie diet.	

Longevity: Lignans that are converted to enterolactone and enterodiole were found to reduce risk of death from all causes.

Migraine headache: Magnesium relaxes muscles and nerves and is often low in migraine sufferers.

PMS symptoms: Magnesium reduces symptoms including moodiness, bloating, and headaches.

Pregnancy: Folate protects against a number of congenital malformations, including neural tube birth defects.

Stroke: Eating a diet rich in whole grains was found to lower risk of stroke.

Type 2 diabetes: Higher intakes of whole grains are associated with increased sensitivity to insulin.

Weight loss and weight control: Fiber-containing foods provide a feeling of fullness; fiber slows digestion, helping to keep blood sugar levels stable and reduce insulin spikes that can trigger cravings and encourage fat storage.

HEALTH SPOTLIGHT

Millet May Help Prevent Gallstones

Millet contains insoluble fiber associated with reduced risk of gallstones. In a study published in the *American Journal of Gastroenterology* that tracked the fiber intake of 69,000 women over a sixteen-year period, those who consumed the most insoluble fiber in whole grains such as millet had a 17 percent lower risk of developing gallstones. It could be because insoluble fiber speeds the time it takes for food to travel through the intestines while reducing bile acid secretion (which can lead to gallstones).

QUICK TIPS

❖ Serve millet in place of rice or potatoes as a side dish. For millet that's more like rice, leave the lid on while cooking; for creamier millet, leave the lid off, stir frequently, and add a little more liquid.

❖ Try millet instead of oatmeal for breakfast; top with honey or agave, dried fruit, bananas, or soymilk.

Millet Hash

2 cups water

1 cup millet

$^1/_4$ cup oyster sauce

2 tablespoons sherry

$^1/_4$ cup plus 2 tablespoons safflower oil

2 teaspoons toasted sesame oil

2 tablespoons minced ginger

3 cloves garlic, minced

1 small carrot, diced

4 ounces shiitake mushrooms, sliced

1 baby bok choy, thinly sliced

4 ounces cooked bay shrimp

4 ounces cooked ham, diced

4 scallions, green and white parts,
sliced on bias into 1-inch pieces

4 ounces sugar snap peas

Bring the water to a boil in a medium saucepan. Add the millet to the boiling water. Turn the heat to very low, cover, and allow the millet to cook for 20 to 25 minutes until all the water has been absorbed. Allow the cooked millet to cool.

Combine the oyster sauce and the sherry. Set aside for later use.

In a large skillet, over low heat, warm 2 tablespoons of the safflower oil with 1 teaspoon of the sesame oil. Add the ginger and the garlic. Heat, stirring constantly, until the herbs are soft and fragrant. Turn heat up and add the carrots, mushrooms, and baby bok choy. Cook over medium heat, stirring frequently, until the bok choy is just wilted. Remove vegetables from the skillet and set aside for later use. Wipe the skillet clean with a paper towel. On high, heat the remaining $^1/_4$ cup of safflower oil with 1 teaspoon of sesame oil in the pan. Add the cooled millet to the hot oil. Allow the millet to brown in spots, turning every now and then until the oil is completely absorbed. Turn heat to low. Add the vegetables back into the pan. Add the shrimp, ham, scallions, and peas. Pour the oyster sauce/sherry mixture over the millet and turn just to coat. Serve.

30. MISO

This fermented soybean paste from Japan is considered a condiment, but miso offers much more than flavor. Often made into miso soup, it provides protein and vitamin B_{12}, along with essential minerals like manganese, zinc, and copper. Miso is also high in tryptophan, so it promotes relaxation and sleep. And because it's fermented, it is a good source of healthy bacteria, which like yogurt, benefits digestion. One warning—miso is high in sodium, so use it in moderation.

HEALTH BENEFITS

Research shows compounds and nutrients found in miso may benefit:

Anemia: Miso contains iron, which can prevent anemia that leads to fatigue, leg cramps, and difficulty concentrating.

Antioxidant defense: Manganese is a cofactor in the production of enzymes important in squelching free radicals.

Anxiety: Tryptophan is necessary for the synthesis of the feel-good chemical serotonin that helps regulate anxiety and mood.

Breast cancer: Miso is associated with a reduced risk (see Health Spotlight).

Depression: Low levels of vitamin B_{12} can contribute to depression.

Diabetes: Manganese may help prevent glucose intolerance that leads to diabetes.

Energy: Copper and manganese are essential components of the enzyme super-oxide dismutase (SOD), which is important in energy production; vitamin B_{12} promotes energy.

Fibromyalgia: Manganese is important for healthy nerve function and may benefit fibromyalgia.

Healthy hair and skin: Copper is necessary to produce melanin for healthy hair color, as well as in forming collagen for youthful skin.

Heart disease: Copper helped prevent heart failure in a study; vitamin B_{12} benefits high homocysteine levels that can lead to heart disease.

Immunity: Zinc promotes immune-cell activity; even a mild deficiency can impair immune function and increase susceptibility to infections.

Insomnia: Tryptophan is a precursor for serotonin, a neurotransmitter that regulates sleep.

Irritable bowel syndrome: Miso provides healthy bacteria plus fiber to benefit symptoms including gas, pain, and bloating.

Osteoporosis: Copper is essential for the formation of collagen, a major protein that makes up bone; manganese and calcium are also required for the synthesis of bone; vitamin K plays an important role in bone health.

PMS symptoms: Manganese and calcium help relieve cramps and other premenstrual symptoms.

Prostate health: Zinc is concentrated in the prostate; low levels are linked to a higher risk of prostate cancer.

Varicose veins: Copper helps promote blood vessel flexibility.

Wound healing: Manganese activates an enzyme that helps form collagen.

MISO NUTRITION INFORMATION

Serving Size 1 ounce (about 2 tablespoons) miso

Amount Per Serving

Calories 56	Calories from fat 14

	% Daily Value
Total Fat 2 grams	3%
Saturated fat 0 gm	0%
Trans fat 0 gm	†
Cholesterol 0 milligrams	0%
Sodium 1,044 mg	43%
Total Carbohydrate 7 gm	2%
Dietary fiber 2 gm	6%
Sugars 2 gm	†
Protein 3 gm	6%
Vitamin A	0%
Vitamin C	0%
Calcium	2%
Iron	4%
Also contains:	
Manganese	12%
Vitamin K	10%
Copper	6%
Zinc	5%
Vitamin B_{12} (cobalamin)	4%

† Daily Value not established.
* Percent Daily Values are based on a 2,000-calorie diet.

HEALTH SPOTLIGHT

Miso May Cut Risk of Breast Cancer

In Japan, higher consumption of fermented soybean foods like miso correlates with lower incidences of breast cancer. With this in mind, scientists fed lab rats either miso or a control diet without miso. They found that miso delayed the appearance of breast cancer compared with the control group. The miso group also had a higher number of benign tumors. Based on these results, the researchers concluded that miso consumption may be a factor in the lower incidences of breast cancer in Japanese women.

QUICK TIPS

❖ Try instant miso soup packets—just add hot water and enjoy. You can also make soup by adding miso paste to hot water. Add sliced fresh shiitake mushrooms (page 186) if desired. This is an excellent soup if you are sick—both miso and shiitake boost the immune system.

❖ Miso can be used in place of salt in many recipes.

Stir-Fried Eggplant in Miso Sauce

YIELD: 6 SERVINGS

$1^1/_2$ pounds baby eggplant, diced into $^1/_4$-inch cubes

3 tablespoons salt

$^1/_4$ cup mirin

$^1/_4$ cup soy sauce

$^1/_4$ cup honey

$^1/_4$ cup sake

$^1/_4$ cup rice vinegar

$^1/_2$ cup toasted sesame oil

1 to 3 dry Japanese peppers, crushed

2 tablespoons fresh minced ginger

3 cloves garlic, minced

1 pound boneless, skinless chicken breast,
cubed into 1-inch pieces

6 large shiitake mushrooms,
each sliced into 3 pieces

$1/4$ cup plus 2 tablespoons shiro (white) miso

6 scallions, green and white parts,
cut into 1-inch pieces

6 servings brown rice or buckwheat noodles
prepared according to package directions

Liberally salt the eggplant and allow it to sit while you make the sauce. In a small bowl, whisk well to combine the mirin, soy sauce, honey, sake, and rice vinegar. Set aside for later use.

Discard any liquid that may have come off the eggplant and collected in the bowl. Rinse the eggplant to wash away all the salt. Allow the eggplant to drain completely before cooking it.

In a very large skillet, over a high flame, heat the sesame oil until the surface begins to ripple. Add the crushed pepper, ginger, and garlic. Cook, stirring constantly, just until the mixture becomes very fragrant. Add the cubed chicken. Continue to cook over high heat stirring frequently until the chicken is no longer pink. Add the eggplant and mushrooms. Continue to cook over high heat, stirring frequently for about 8 minutes. Add the mirin/soy sauce/honey/sake/vinegar mixture to the pan and continue to cook over high heat for 2 more minutes. Turn the heat to low. Move the vegetables and chicken to one side of the pan, leaving the sauce on the other. Whisk the miso into the sauce. Toss the chicken and vegetables in the miso sauce to completely coat. Stir in the scallions. Serve over brown rice or buckwheat noodles.

31. OATS

"You have to eat oatmeal or you'll dry up.
Anybody knows that."
—KAY THOMPSON (1908–1998), COMPOSER, ACTRESS,
AND AUTHOR OF THE *ELOISE* CHILDREN'S BOOKS

The ancient Greeks elevated oats to dessert status, while the Romans regarded oats as fit only for animal fodder. If only they had known the many benefits of eating oats! Oats not only supply "good carbs," protein, and both soluble and insoluble fiber, but they are high in minerals and amino acids including selenium, tryptophan, manganese, phosphorus, and thiamine as well. Plus, phytonutrient phenolics in oats act as antioxidants, much like those found in fruits and vegetables. The soluble fiber beta-glucan in oatmeal boosts immunity and combats diabetes. And oats contain phytoestrogens, plant compounds that may combat breast cancer and heart disease, and keep bones strong. All this in one bowl of breakfast cereal! Let's be honest, though—that grey clump of oatmeal can be a little boring. Try the recipes here for oatmeal that you'll actually look forward to in the morning.

HEALTH BENEFITS

Research shows compounds and nutrients found in oats may benefit:

Alzheimer's disease: Phenolics may protect brain cells from damage.

Anxiety: Women with social anxiety disorder who took thiamine were more clear-headed and composed.

Asthma: Eating a diet that includes plenty of whole grains was found to cut the risk of childhood asthma by 50 percent; selenium may also decrease symptoms.

Breast cancer: Phytoestrogens may be protective, possibly by blocking the development of estrogen-related cancer; a high-fiber diet decreases risk.

Cataracts: Thiamine—along with other nutrients—shows promise in lowering the risk of developing cataracts; phenolics may also add protection.

Colon cancer: Eating a diet high in whole grains was found to lower the risk of colon cancer, possibly because insoluble fiber moves harmful toxins and cancer-causing substances out of the colon more quickly.

Digestive health: Fiber improves digestion and is linked to a reduced risk of hemorrhoids and diverticulitis (bulging tissue pouches in the colon); thiamine aids in production of hydrochloric acid (which is necessary for proper digestion).

Energy: Manganese is a component of superoxide dismutase (SOD), an enzyme that's essential in energy production.

Heart disease: Phenolic antioxidants called avenanthramides, found only in oats, help prevent LDL cholesterol damage that can lead to atherosclerosis; lignans benefit heart health by binding bile and blood cholesterol together and helping to shuttle it out of the body.

High blood pressure: Whole grains including oats have been shown to keep blood pressure down.

High cholesterol: Beta-glucan and fiber help reduce cholesterol (see Heart Disease).

OATS NUTRITION INFORMATION

Serving Size 1/4 cup steel-cut oats, dry

Amount Per Serving

Calories 150 — Calories from fat 20

	% Daily Value*
Total Fat 2 grams	3%
Saturated fat 0 gm	0%
Trans fat 0 gm	†
Cholesterol 0 milligrams	0%
Sodium 0 mg	0%
Total Carbohydrate 26 gm	9%
Dietary fiber 4 gm	15%
Sugars 0 gm	†
Protein 4 gm	8%
Vitamin A	0%
Vitamin C	0%
Calcium	2%
Iron	6%
Also contains:	
Manganese	74%
Selenium	15%
Phosphorus	15%
Vitamin B_1 (thiamine)	12%

† Daily Value not established.

* Percent Daily Values are based on a 2,000-calorie diet.

Immunity: Beta-glucan boosts the immune system's response to infection.

Insomnia: Tryptophan is a precursor for serotonin, a neurotransmitter that regulates sleep.

Osteoporosis: Phytoestrogens, manganese, and phosphorus help keep bones strong.

Type 2 diabetes: Beta-glucan and fiber-rich foods help slow the release of glucose into the bloodstream; magnesium helps lower blood sugar and is thought to lower diabetes risk.

HEALTH SPOTLIGHT

A Second Look at Oatmeal and Cholesterol

In 1997, the Food and Drug Administration (FDA) granted companies the right to label packaging with the claim that oatmeal "lowers cholesterol." This landmark decision was based on the convincing body of evidence available at the time. More recently, a 2009 report examining subsequent research shows even greater support for oatmeal's cholesterol-lowering abilities than previously thought. The report states that follow-up studies unanimously confirm that oats reduce total cholesterol levels, and moreover, lower harmful low-density lipoprotein (LDL) cholesterol without adversely affecting healthy high-density lipoprotein (HDL) cholesterol or triglycerides.

QUICK TIP

❖ Instant oatmeal is easier, but it's been processed so that the beneficial bran and germ have been removed, plus it usually contains added sugars. Steel-cut oats can be almost as easy if you pre-measure and soak them overnight in a saucepan in the refrigerator. Before soaking, bring the water to a boil then add the oats. Cover and refrigerate. In the morning, just bring to a boil and simmer, uncovered, stirring occasionally as you go about your routine. Your oatmeal will be ready in about 10 minutes. For toppings try: berries (fresh or dried), honey, cinnamon, wheat germ, or chopped nuts.

Oatmeal Three Ways

Pumpkin Oatmeal

$1/_4$ cup steel-cut oats

1 cup unsweetened soymilk

$1/_2$ cup canned pumpkin

Pinch salt

2 tablespoons agave nectar

In a medium saucepan, over very low heat, heat the oats and soymilk. Cook uncovered, stirring often for 25 to 30 minutes. Add the pumpkin, salt, and agave. Increase the heat to medium. Cook, stirring constantly, until desired consistency. Serve immediately.

Orange Oatmeal

1 cup unsweetened soymilk

1 Earl Grey tea bag

$1/_4$ cup steel-cut oats

$1/_4$ cup thawed orange juice concentrate

2 teaspoons sucanat

1 teaspoon vanilla extract

Pinch salt

In a medium saucepan, over medium heat, scald the soymilk (heat to just below boiling). Remove from the heat and steep the teabag in the hot soymilk for 3 minutes. Remove and discard the teabag. Add the oats to the soymilk and cook the mixture over very low heat, uncovered, for 25 to 30 minutes, stirring often, until most of the liquid has been absorbed. Add the orange juice concentrate, sucanat, vanilla, and salt. Stir constantly, over medium heat, until you have desired consistency. Serve immediately.

Chocolate-Chai Oatmeal

1 cup unsweetened soymilk

1 chai tea bag

$^1/_4$ cup steel-cut oats

1 ounce dark (70% or darker) chocolate,
finely chopped

$^1/_4$ cup dried, unsweetened coconut

1 teaspoon vanilla extract

Pinch salt

In a medium saucepan, over medium heat, scald the soymilk (heat to just below boiling). Remove from the heat and steep the teabag for 3 minutes. Remove and discard the teabag. Add the oats. Cook over very low heat, uncovered, stirring frequently, 25 to 30 minutes until most of the liquid has been absorbed. Remove from the heat. Stir in the chocolate, coconut, vanilla, and salt. Serve immediately.

*   *   *

For other recipes and ways of using oats, see: Blueberry Quick Bread (page 56), Goji Berry Granola (107), Whole-Wheat Maple Schmootz Muffins (page 119), Muesli (page 220).

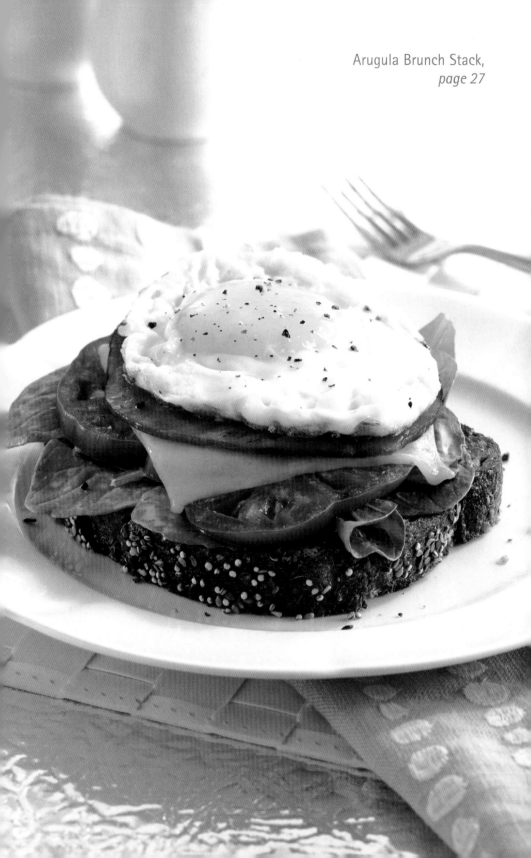

Arugula Brunch Stack,
page 27

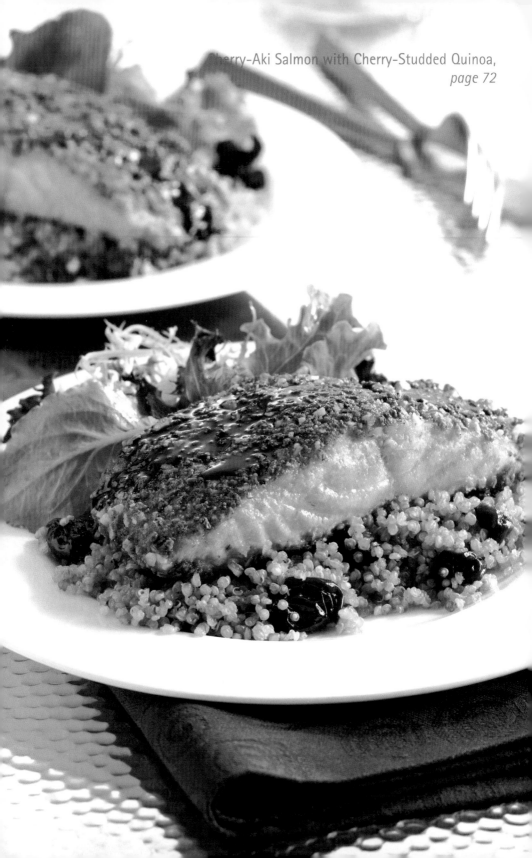

Cherry-Aki Salmon with Cherry-Studded Quinoa,
page 72

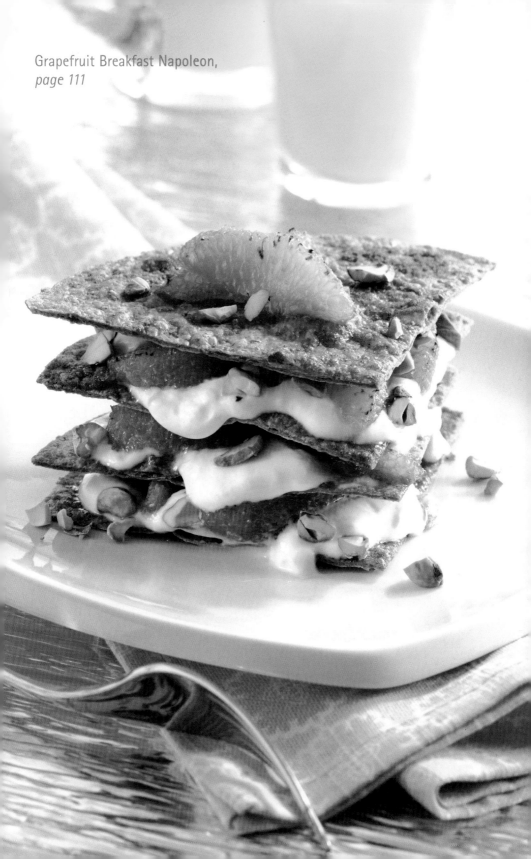

Grapefruit Breakfast Napoleon,
page 111

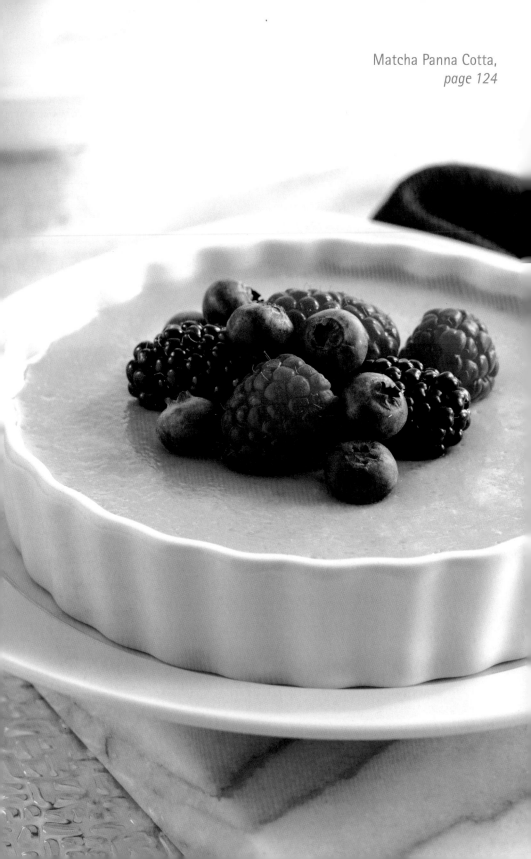

Matcha Panna Cotta,
page 124

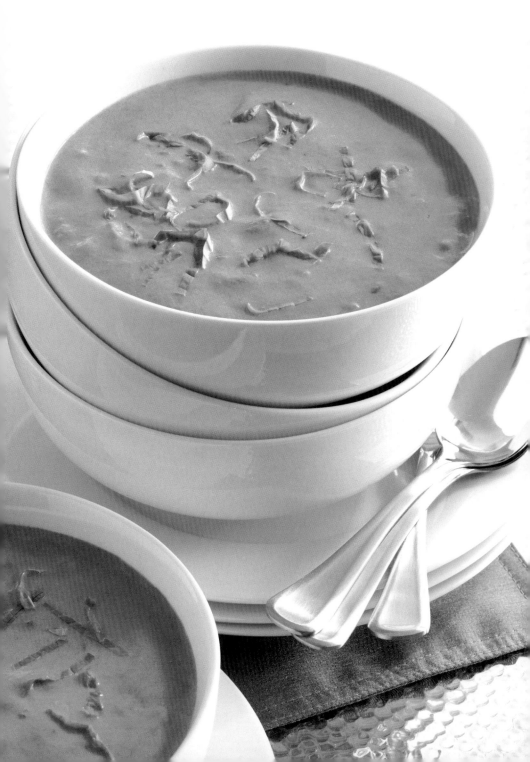

Pumpkin Potage,
page 164

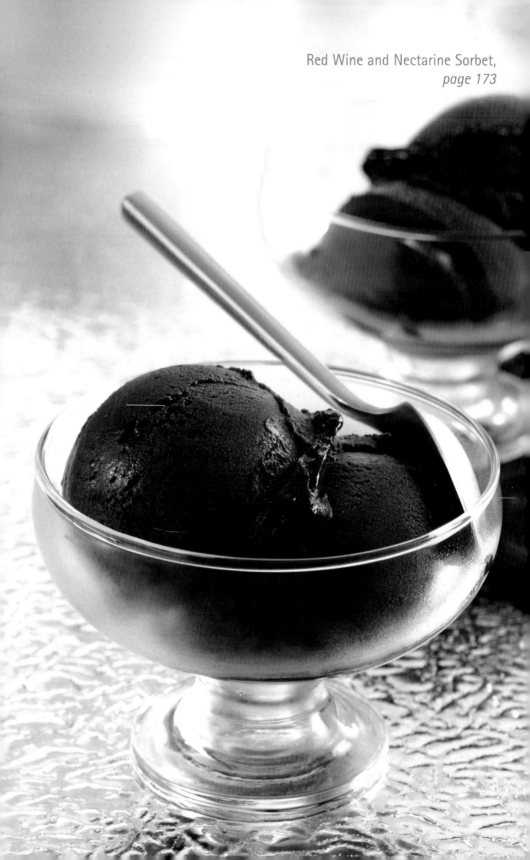

Red Wine and Nectarine Sorbet, *page 173*

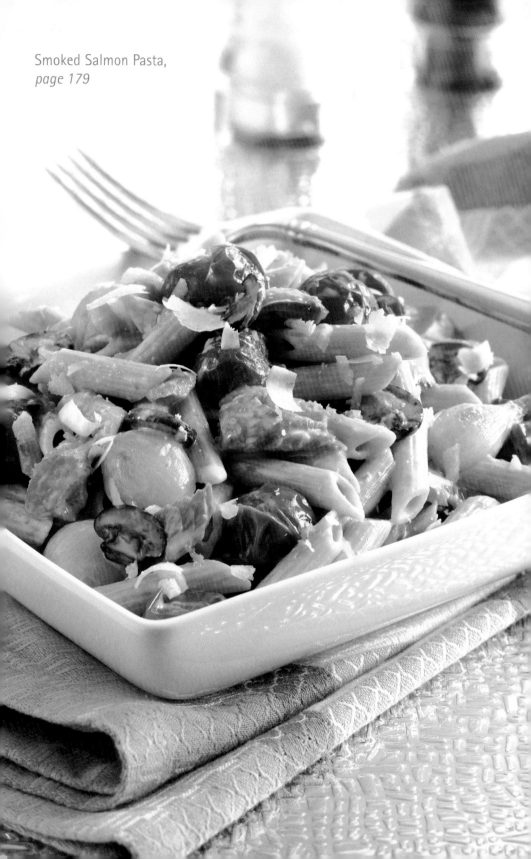

Smoked Salmon Pasta,
page 179

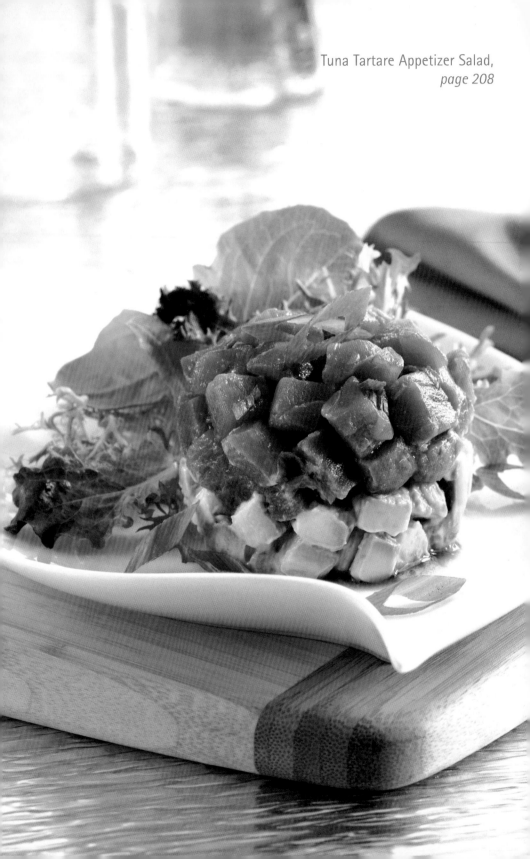

Tuna Tartare Appetizer Salad,
page 208

32. OLIVES

Olives have a rich history, appearing in ancient Greek mythology and in Egyptian art, and have long been associated with peace and wisdom. They are native to the Mediterranean, and have been cultivated since 3,000 B.C. Olives contain 75 percent oleic acid, the monounsaturated fat also present in olive oil, and are rich in antioxidant polyphenols and flavonoids, which, along with monounsaturated fat, help protect cells and reduce inflammation. The maslinic acid in their skin defends against colon cancer. And the polyphenol hydroxytyrosol and vitamin E in olives deter heart disease. The many varieties of olives range in flavor from slightly sweet and fruity to salty and briny, and offer great gastronomy to Greek, Italian, and Spanish cuisines. Black olives are fully ripe, while green olives have been harvested early, but there are no significant nutritional differences between the two.

HEALTH BENEFITS

Research shows compounds and nutrients found in olives may benefit:

Attention deficit/hyperactivity disorder: Low levels of omega-3 and omega-9 fatty acids are associated with ADHD.

Alzheimer's disease: Vitamin E is reported to slow down cognitive decline in people with Alzheimer's (see Health Spotlight).

Asthma: Vitamin E, monounsaturated fats, and polyphenols decrease inflammation and may be effective in reducing severity of pain and increasing joint function.

Brain health: Hydroxytyrosol shows promise in protecting brain cells.

Breast cancer: Diets rich in monounsaturated fat are linked to lower risk of breast cancer.

Cell and DNA protection: Vitamin E and other antioxidants may prevent free-radical damage to cell membranes and DNA.

Colon cancer: Maslinic acid protects against colon cancer; higher intakes of monounsaturated fats are linked to lower risk.

Energy: Olive oil helps protect the mitochondria (energy-producing part of the cell) from oxidative damage.

Heart disease: Studies suggest hydroxytyrosol and vitamin E prevent free-radical damage to blood vessels that can lead to heart disease.

High cholesterol: Oleic acid may inhibit LDL (bad) cholesterol from oxidizing and damaging blood vessels.

Hot flashes: Studies show vitamin E is an effective treatment for hot flashes.

Immunity: Oleic acid may be necessary for healthy immune system function.

Osteo- and rheumatoid arthritis: Vitamin E, monounsaturated fats, and polyphenols decrease inflammation and may be effective in reducing pain and increasing joint function.

Osteoporosis: Low levels of fatty acids such as omega-3 and omega-9 are associated with greater bone loss.

OLIVES NUTRITION INFORMATION

Serving Size 1 ounce (about 8) green olives

Amount Per Serving

Calories 41	Calories from fat 36

	% Daily Value*
Total Fat 4 grams	7%
Saturated fat 1 gm	3%
Trans fat 0 gm	†
Cholesterol 0 milligrams	0%
Sodium 436 mg	18%
Total Carbohydrate 1 gm	.33%
Dietary fiber 1 gm	4%
Sugars 0 gm	†
Protein 0 gm	0%
Vitamin A	2%
Vitamin C	0%
Calcium	1%
Iron	1%
Also contains:	
Vitamin E	5%
Copper	2%
Omega-6 fatty acids 30.4 mg	†
Omega-3 fatty acids 2.3 mg	†

† Daily Value not established.
* Percent Daily Values are based on a 2,000-calorie diet.

HEALTH SPOTLIGHT

Part of an Anti-Alzheimer's Disease Diet

Olives contain vitamin E (20 percent of the recommended Daily Value per cup), shown to slow down cognitive decline in Alzheimer's disease patients. A study analyzed Alzheimer's patients taking prescribed Alzheimer's disease drugs. In addition to the prescribed treatment, one group took both vitamin E and an anti-inflammatory, another group took vitamin E but no anti-inflammatory, a third group took an anti-inflammatory but no vitamin E, and a fourth group took neither. After three years, patients taking vitamin E exhibited a slowing of the typical decline seen in cognitive function of Alzheimer's disease patients.

QUICK TIPS

❖ Blue-cheese stuffed green olives make a fantastic snack or appetizer.

❖ Use olives liberally on pizza and in pasta and salads.

Tapenade

YIELD: APPROXIMATELY 2 CUPS

1 bulb garlic

4 tablespoons olive oil

1 large shallot, minced

1 cup whole Kalamata olives, minced

$1/4$ cup sundried tomatoes packed in oil, minced

$1/3$ cup pine nuts, minced

1 tablespoon minced fresh oregano

$1/3$ cup feta cheese, crumbled

1 tablespoon fresh squeezed lemon juice

Zest from squeezed lemon

(zest before juicing)

Preheat oven to 350°F.

Slice just enough off the top of the garlic bulb to reveal the cloves. Place the bulb in the center of a square of aluminum foil. Pour 2 tablespoons of the olive oil over the top of the bulb. Fold the foil so that you create an envelope around the bulb and oil. Bake for 40 minutes. Allow the bulb to cool completely. Remove the softened cloves from the papery skin by squeezing each clove. Mince the cloves.

In a small skillet, over very low heat, caramelize the minced shallot in the remaining 2 tablespoons of olive oil, just until they start to take on color. This should be a long, slow process and can be done while the garlic is roasting. Allow the shallots to cool completely. Do not discard the olive oil. Include it in the tapenade when you add the shallots.

In a medium bowl, combine the roasted garlic, caramelized shallots (with the oil), olives, sundried tomatoes, pine nuts, oregano, feta, lemon juice, and zest. Mix well.

Serve as an appetizer on crostini or as a sandwich spread.

* * *

For other recipes and ways of using olives, see: Quinoa-Chicken Salad (page 169).

33. ONIONS

In ancient Egypt, onions were so highly revered they were used as currency, and even placed in King Tut's tomb for him to carry with him to the afterlife. In India, onions have been used as medicine for centuries. In the United States today, onions are a common ingredient in chicken soup, helping to fight the common cold with high amounts of vitamin C plus antibacterial compounds. Onions are rich in chromium, potassium, fiber, tryptophan, folate, and flavonoids including quercetin and kaempferol—giving onions strong anti-cancer activity. A member of the allium family (like garlic), onions contain sulfur compounds that give them powerful health-protective properties (these compounds are also what cause tears when chopping). Varieties differ when it comes to content of beneficial phytonutrients, phenols, and flavonoids. For example, shallots have the most phenols and are the highest in antioxidants, while the Western yellow onion contains the most flavonoids. The caramelized onion recipe here uses white onions, a sweet variety high in vitamin C and a source of quercetin.

HEALTH BENEFITS

Research shows compounds and nutrients found in onions may benefit:

Anxiety: Tryptophan increases the mood-boosting chemical serotonin and promotes relaxation.

Asthma: Onions contain an abundance of anti-inflammatory compounds that reduce inflammatory conditions including asthma.

Atherosclerosis: Onions may reduce stickiness of blood platelets.

Breast cancer: Quercetin and other flavonoids have been shown to inhibit the growth of breast cancer cells; onions are associated with a 25 percent reduced risk of breast cancer.

Colon cancer: Quercetin was found to stop tumor growth and protect cells.

Common cold: Quercetin plus vitamin C boosts the immune system to fend off colds.

Depression: Low levels of folate are linked to depression.

Heart disease: Studies show quercetin and other flavonoids may lower heart disease risk by up to 20 percent.

High blood pressure: Eating a diet that includes plenty of sulfur-containing vegetables (also rich in flavonoids and chromium) like onions has been shown to lower high blood pressure.

High cholesterol: Regular consumption of onions has been shown to lower cholesterol.

Insomnia: Tryptophan is a precursor for serotonin, a neurotransmitter that regulates sleep.

Longevity: Antioxidants help protect against the formation of free radicals, which promote aging and disease.

ONIONS NUTRITION INFORMATION		
Serving Size 1 large onion (about 1 cup chopped)		
Amount Per Serving		
Calories 64		Calories from fat 1
		% Daily Value*
Total Fat 0 grams		0%
Saturated fat 0 gm		0%
Trans fat 0 gm		†
Cholesterol 0 milligrams		0%
Sodium 6 mg		.25%
Total Carbohydrate 15 gm		5%
Dietary fiber 3 gm		11%
Sugars 7 gm		†
Protein 2 gm		4%
Vitamin A		0%
Vitamin C		20%
Calcium		4%
Iron		2%
Also contains:		
Chromium		20%
Vitamin B_6 (pyridoxine)		10%
Manganese		10%
Folate		8%
Potassium		7%
† Daily Value not established.		
* Percent Daily Values are based on a 2,000-calorie diet.		

Osteo- and rheumatoid arthritis: Several compounds in onions decrease inflammation and may be effective in reducing pain and increasing joint function.

Osteoporosis: A compound in onions called amma-glutamyl peptide prevents osteoclasts (a type of bone cell) from breaking down bone.

Ovarian cancer: Women whose diets were high in kaempferol-containing foods benefited from a 40 percent reduction in ovarian cancer risk.

PMS symptoms: Studies show tryptophan decreases mood swings and irritability.

Prostate cancer: Onion consumption is linked to a 71 percent reduced risk of prostate cancer.

Stroke: Sulfur, chromium, and vitamin B_6 help convert homocysteine (a significant risk factor for stroke) into benign components.

Type 2 diabetes: Chromium helps regulate glucose levels by increasing insulin sensitivity.

HEALTH SPOTLIGHT

Flu Protection

The quercetin in onions may boost immunity and guard against the flu. In a study, mice that performed strenuous exercise (which is thought to increase the risk of upper respiratory infection) were exposed to the flu virus. Those that were given quercetin supplements reduced risk of infection by 63 percent. The researchers' report concluded, "These data suggest that quercetin may prove to be an effective strategy to lessen the impact of stressful exercise on susceptibility to respiratory infection." The same rate of illness was found in mice that did not exercise but were given quercetin, however, suggesting that quercetin can help ward off the flu in non-athletes as well.

QUICK TIPS

❖ For easy low-fat, less-mess onion rings, cut a large brown onion into rings. Dip slices in beaten egg, then coat them in seasoned bread crumbs. Bake the onion rings on a greased baking sheet for about 20 minutes at 400°F.

Worth-the-Wait Caramelized Onion Bruschetta

YIELD: 36 APPETIZERS

4 pounds white onions, thinly sliced

$1/_2$ cup olive oil

4 ounces prosciutto, coarsely chopped

$1/_2$ cup thawed apple juice concentrate

3 tablespoons whole-grain mustard

1 12-inch multigrain baguette,
sliced into 36 pieces

1 cup finely grated extra-sharp cheddar cheese

In a very large skillet, combine the onions and the olive oil. Place over extremely low heat, turning every 15 to 20 minutes until they are soft and golden brown. They should have reduced in volume by about three quarters. This process could take 3 to 4 hours if truly done over a low heat. There should be no liquid left in the pan and the onions should be uniformly brown. At this point, the onions can be refrigerated and then reheated for serving later if desired.

Preheat oven to 350°F.

When there is no liquid left in the pan and the onions are uniformly golden brown, stir in the prosciutto, apple juice concentrate, and mustard. Turn the heat to medium high and stir constantly until the apple juice concentrate has evaporated. Lightly toast the bread slices on a baking sheet, about 4 minutes.

Divide the onion mixture evenly to top each slice of bread. Sprinkle lightly with the grated extra-sharp cheddar cheese. Serve immediately.

*   *   *

For other recipes and ways of using onions, see: Scallops in Almond-Herb Sauce (page 10), Roasted Pork Tenderloin with Apple-Brie Sauce (page 19), Apricot Moroccan-Style Stew (page 23), Creamy Asparagus Soup (page 33), Avocado-Tuna Wraps (page 37), Black Bean Falafel (page 51), Dad's Braised Green Cabbage (page 65), Black Bean Burritos with Spicy Chili Salsa (page

77), Coffee-Braised Pork Loin (page 82), Cucumber Relish (page 87), Mussels in Fennel Broth (page 100), Mango and Herb Pasta with Peanut Sauce (page 115), Millet Hash (page 129), Stir-Fried Eggplant in Miso Sauce (page 132), Earl Grey-Orange Chicken (page 151), Pineapple Salsa on Shrimp Patties (page 155), Quinoa Quick Tips (page 168), Quinoa-Chicken Salad (page 169), Smoked Salmon Pasta (page 179), Spinach Salad with Whole-Wheat Toast Points (page 190), Tomato-Seafood Chowder (page 203), Tuna Tartare Appetizer Salad (page 208), Macadamia-Pineapple Curry (page 213).

34. ORANGES

Oranges are known to be an abundant source of vitamin C, but present in about the same amounts, oranges also contain phytonutrient compounds called limonoids that act as powerful anti-carcinogens against cancer and remain active in the body up to twenty-four hours after consumption. It is these limonoids that give oranges their unique aroma, the fragrance of which has been shown to decrease violent and aggressive behavior. All in all, oranges are loaded with 170 phytochemicals and 60 flavonoids that help defend against disease, including nobiletin, tangeretin, and limonin. One particular flavanone in oranges, hesperidin (found primarily in the rind and white pulp), is emerging as a star component, showing promise in heart health and as an anti-inflammatory. The recipe here for Earl Grey-Orange Chicken features oranges along with orange zest (a good source of hesperidin).

HEALTH BENEFITS

Research shows compounds and nutrients found in oranges may benefit:

Alzheimer's disease: Citrus flavanones may offer neuroprotection.

Asthma: Vitamin C reduces inflammation that can restrict airways.

Cancer: Studies show limonoids can help fight cancers of the stomach, skin, mouth, lung, breast, and colon; mandarin oranges showed significant benefit in liver cancer; also beneficial is beta-cryptoxanthin (a carotenoid found in yellow and orange fruits and vegetables), which was found to be protective against lung cancer.

Cataracts: Eating a diet that includes plenty of citrus fruits was found effective in reducing risk of cataracts.

Common cold: Vitamin C boosts immunity and may reduce cold symptoms.

Gingivitis: Vitamin C promotes healing, especially of bleeding gums.

High cholesterol: Tangeretin and nobiletin may lower cholesterol (see Health Spotlight); limonin (a limonoid) may work to lower cholesterol.

Kidney stones: Orange juice was found to increase citric acid excretion in the urine, decreasing the likelihood of forming stones.

Lung cancer: Consuming foods rich in beta-cryptoxanthin may lower lung cancer risk.

Macular degeneration (age-related): Eating three or more servings of fruit a day is linked to decreased risk.

Osteoarthritis: Vitamin C reduces inflammation and free-radical damage within joints; it is also essential for production and maintenance of collagen, a major protein found in cartilage that helps cushion joints.

Parkinson's disease: Tangeretin may offer neuroprotective effects.

ORANGES NUTRITION INFORMATION

Serving Size 1 orange, raw (about 1 cup)

Amount Per Serving

Calories 107	Calories from fat 4

	% Daily Value*
Total Fat 1 grams	1%
Saturated fat 0 gm	0%
Trans fat 0 gm	†
Cholesterol 0 milligrams	0%
Sodium 3 mg	.125%
Total Carbohydrate 26 gm	9%
Dietary fiber 8 gm	31%
Sugars 0 gm	†
Protein 2 gm	4%
Vitamin A	8%
Vitamin C	201%
Calcium	12%
Iron	8%

Also contains:

Vitamin B$_1$ (thiamine)	11%

† Daily Value not established.
* Percent Daily Values are based on a 2,000-calorie diet.

Prostate cancer: Naringenin has been shown to help repair damaged DNA in the prostate.

Rheumatoid arthritis: A glass of fresh squeezed orange juice a day decreased risk of developing rheumatoid arthritis by up to 52 percent, attributed to compounds zeaxanthin and cryptoxanthin.

Skin health: Vitamin C aids in collagen formation and protects against free-radical damage.

Stroke: Studies found an association between citrus fruit juice consumption and lowered ischemic stroke risk.

Type 2 diabetes: Fiber helps control blood sugar levels by slowing the release of glucose into the bloodstream.

Ulcers: Oranges appear to prevent infection from *H. pylori,* the bacteria responsible for the development of peptic ulcers; this, in turn, could prevent stomach cancer.

Weight loss and weight control: Fiber-containing foods provide a feeling of fullness; fiber slows digestion, helping to keep blood sugar levels stable and reduce insulin spikes that can trigger cravings and encourage fat storage.

HEALTH SPOTLIGHT

More Effective Than Drugs at Lowering Cholesterol

Orange zest contains the polymethoxylated flavones (PMFs) tangeretin and nobiletin, which a study showed may lower cholesterol better than some prescription drugs. In the study, diet-induced high LDL (bad) cholesterol was lowered by up to 40 percent after ingestion of these flavones. Meanwhile, HDL (good) cholesterol was not affected—and there were no negative side effects. The findings were published in the May 2004 issue of *Journal of Agricultural and Food Chemistry.*

QUICK TIPS

❖ Add an orange slice to a cup of green tea. A new study shows citrus increases the antioxidant power of catechins in green tea.

❖ Choose juice over vitamin water. Researchers found that real orange juice fortified with vitamin C protected DNA against free-radical damage, whereas plain water fortified with vitamin C did not. They speculate that the phytochemicals in the juice, including flavanones and carotenoids, work together in yet-to-be-fully-understood ways to provide antioxidant protection.

Earl Grey-Orange Chicken

YIELD: 6 SERVINGS

Sauce

$1/4$ cup soy sauce

$1/2$ cup plus 2 tablespoons rice vinegar

1 cup fresh squeezed orange juice

2 tablespoons cane sugar

$1/2$ ounce or $1/4$ cup loose Earl Grey tea

Chicken

2 pounds boneless, skinless chicken (breast or thigh),
cut into 1-inch cubes

Salt and pepper

3 tablespoons vegetable oil

1 tablespoon finely grated ginger

1 tablespoon finely minced garlic

1 small Thai chili, seeded, membranes removed, sliced

$1/2$ cup thinly sliced scallions, green and white parts

2 oranges, supremed (see directions on page 47)

Slurry

1 teaspoon xanthan gum*

1 tablespoon toasted sesame oil

1 tablespoon finely grated orange zest

Salt and pepper

2 oranges, supremed
(zest oranges before making the supreme)

* If xanthan gum is unavailable, you can thicken the sauce with a cornstarch slurry.
Dissolve 2 teaspoons of cornstarch in 2 tablespoons of cold liquid, creating a slurry.
You could use a little extra orange juice for this. Add the cornstarch slurry when you
add the sesame oil and the orange zest. Whisk well. Cook to thicken.

TO MAKE THE SAUCE: In a small saucepan, combine the soy sauce, rice
vinegar, orange juice, and cane sugar. Bring the mixture just to a simmer.
Turn off the heat and add the tea. Steep it in the orange juice mixture
for 5 minutes. Strain out and discard the tea.

TO MAKE THE CHICKEN: Lightly season the chicken with salt and pepper. Heat the vegetable oil in a large skillet. Stir-fry the chicken until it is no longer visibly pink. The chicken will not be fully cooked yet. Add the ginger, garlic, chili, and scallions to the pan. Continue to cook, stirring constantly until the garlic and ginger are fragrant, about 2 more minutes. Be careful not to brown the garlic. Next, supreme the oranges. Add the sauce and orange supremes to the skillet. Simmer to reduce the sauce and complete cooking of the chicken, about 5 minutes.

TO MAKE THE SLURRY: Dissolve the xanthan gum in the sesame oil to create a slurry. Whisk the xanthan gum slurry and orange zest into the sauce. Cook, stirring constantly, until the sauce thickens, about 2 more minutes. Serve immediately over brown rice.

* * *

For other recipes and ways of using oranges and orange zest, see: Cranberry-Chocolate Tart (page 5), Roasted Beet and Fennel Salad (page 45), Orange Oatmeal (page 137), Smoked Salmon Pasta (page 179).

35. PINEAPPLE

It's more than just a sweet addition to your piña colada. South American Guarani Indians called the pineapple *nana* (translated to mean "excellent fruit"). We have to agree. Loaded with vitamins and minerals and high in fiber, pineapple is not only delicious but nutritious as well. Fresh pineapple—not canned—contains an anti-inflammatory enzyme called bromelain that has been credited in easing arthritis pain and stiffness, decreasing muscle soreness, and relieving bruising. Although concentrated in the stem, bromelain is present in the fruit in lesser quantities. It is this powerful component that also makes pineapple juice an excellent meat tenderizer and ingredient in marinades.

HEALTH BENEFITS

Research shows compounds and nutrients found in pineapple may benefit:

Allergies and sinusitis: Bromelain can help relieve inflammation and swelling.

Angina: Bromelain has been shown to thin blood and relieve pain associated with angina.

Blood clots: Bromelain appears to act as an anti-coagulant.

Bone health: Manganese is vital for bone formation; a deficiency can cause abnormal skeletal development and bone loss.

Bronchitis and asthma: Bromelain can help loosen mucus.

Bruising: Bromelain may speed healing and reduce inflammation.

Cancer: Bromelain shows promise in fighting cancer, according to some studies; some documented cases show bromelain may cause cancerous tumors to regress.

Coughs: Bromelain may suppress coughs.

Diarrhea: Bromelain helps prevent traveller's diarrhea by preventing *E. coli* bacteria from attaching to intestinal walls.

Digestive health: Bromelain aids overall digestion by helping to break down protein.

Edema: Bromelain has been shown to reduce fluid retention.

High cholesterol: Antioxidants including vitamin C fight free radicals that can promote buildup of cholesterol plaques.

Immunity: Vitamin C enhances the immune system's ability to fight ear infections, colds, and flu.

Leukemia: Bromelain shows promise in treating leukemia.

Lung cancer: Bromelain reduces spread of tumor growth in lung cancer.

Macular degeneration (age-related): Eating three or more servings of fruit such as pineapple a day is linked to decreased risk.

Osteo- and rheumatoid arthritis: Bromelain and vitamin C may alleviate arthritis pain by decreasing inflammation and increasing ease of movement (see Health Spotlight).

Strains, sprains, and minor injuries: Bromelain may reduce inflammation and speed healing.

Ulcerative colitis: Bromelain may relieve associated inflammation.

Urinary tract infections (UTIs): Bromelain can enhance the effectiveness of antibiotics.

PINEAPPLE NUTRITION INFORMATION		
Serving Size 1 cup chopped pineapple, fresh		
Amount Per Serving		
Calories 82		Calories from fat 2
		% Daily Value*
Total Fat 0 grams		0%
Saturated fat 0 gm		0%
Trans fat 0 gm		†
Cholesterol 0 milligrams		0%
Sodium 2 mg		.08%
Total Carbohydrate 22 gm		7%
Dietary fiber 2 gm		31%
Sugars 16 gm		†
Protein 1 gm		2%
Vitamin A		2%
Vitamin C		131%
Calcium		2%
Iron		3%
Also contains:		
Manganese		76%
† Daily Value not established.		
* Percent Daily Values are based on a 2,000-calorie diet.		

HEALTH SPOTLIGHT

Better Than Drugs for Arthritis

In a 2004 study published in *Clinical Rheumatology,* an enzyme formula containing bromelain was pitted against the prescription nonsteroidal anti-inflammatory drug (NSAID) diclofenac (brand names Cataflam and Voltaren) for patients with osteoarthritis of the knee. Results showed that 51 percent of patients receiving enzyme therapy reported improvement in pain and restoration of function, versus just 37 percent of people given the drug. The six-week study involved 103 patients.

QUICK TIP

❖ Use fresh pineapple—not canned—to ensure it contains active enzymes. The canning process destroys beneficial enzymes.

❖ Try grilled fresh pineapple slices drizzled with agave syrup (see page 3).

Pineapple Salsa on Shrimp Patties

YIELD: 6 SERVINGS

Shrimp Patties

2 pounds raw shrimp

1 egg

$1/2$ cup finely crushed whole-grain cracker crumbs

Zest of 1 lime

1 jalapeño pepper, roasted (see directions on page 78),
skinned, seeds and membranes removed, minced

$1/4$ cup minced red onion

2 cloves garlic, minced

$1/4$ teaspoon each: black pepper, ground ginger, cumin,
allspice, nutmeg, paprika, and cinnamon

$1/8$ teaspoon ground cloves

$1/2$ teaspoon salt

Pineapple Salsa

2 cups fresh pineapple, diced into $1/4$-inch cubes

1 pasilla chili, roasted (see directions on page 78),
skinned, seeds and membranes removed, diced

1 tablespoon finely minced fresh ginger

$1/2$ teaspoon fresh thyme leaves

$1/2$ cup grated fresh coconut

$1/4$ cup red onion, diced into $1/4$-inch cubes

2 cloves garlic, minced

1 tablespoon honey

1 to 2 tablespoons lime juice
(more or less to taste)

Salt to taste

Coating

4 ounces unsalted macadamia nuts, finely chopped

$2/3$ cup finely crushed whole-grain cracker crumbs

3 tablespoons grape seed oil, for frying

TO PREPARE THE SHRIMP: Peel and devein the shrimp. In the bowl of a food processor fitted with the chopping blade, combine the shrimp, egg, cracker crumbs, zest, jalapeño pepper, onion, garlic, spices, and salt. Pulse until you have a smooth paste and all the ingredients are evenly distributed. Chill the shrimp mixture until ready to prepare for serving. Meanwhile, prepare the salsa.

TO MAKE THE SALSA: Combine the pineapple, pasilla chili, ginger, thyme, coconut, onion, garlic, honey, and lime juice. Add salt to taste. Mix well and refrigerate until ready to serve.

When you are ready to serve, combine the nuts and coating crumbs in a shallow dish. Divide the shrimp mixture into six equal patties. The patties should be about 1-inch thick. Coat the patties on all sides with the crumb/nut mixture. Over low heat, pan-fry the patties in grape seed oil. The patties should brown lightly on each side and be just set firm in the center. Serve hot with the chilled pineapple salsa.

*   *   *

For other recipes and ways of using fresh pineapple, see: Cherry-Aki Salmon with Cherry-Studded Quinoa (page 72), Macadamia-Pineapple Curry (page 213).

36. POMEGRANATE

The ancient Chinese believed the pomegranate could impart immortality, while Babylonian soldiers chewed the seeds before battle, believing doing so would make them invincible. The pomegranate has been a symbol of fertility throughout history, perhaps because of its many seeds. And as it turns out, pomegranates contain potent antioxidants that impact reproductive health, as well as phytoestrogens, which mimic the estrogens in our own bodies and may benefit symptoms related to menopause and prostate cancer. The pomegranate also contains an abundance of antioxidant polyphenols—more than even red wine. In particular, a compound called punicalagin, which accounts for about half the antioxidant power of pomegranates, contributes free-radical scavenging and disease-fighting abilities. In fact, pomegranate juice was ranked "healthiest fruit juice" in a 2008 University of California, Los Angeles (UCLA), study.

HEALTH BENEFITS

Research shows compounds and nutrients found in pomegranates may benefit:

Alzheimer's disease: Pomegranate juice may reduce harmful proteins that lead to Alzheimer's disease, possibly due to the action of polyphenols.

Arthritis: Pomegranate fruit extract appears to block enzymes that contribute to loss of cartilage; pomegranate juice helps reduce inflammation.

Bone loss (menopause-related): Phytoestrogens may help prohibit bone loss.

Breast cancer: Polyphenols appear to block the synthesis of estrogen and inhibit the growth of breast cancer cells.

Depression (menopause-related): Phytoestrogens may improve depression associated with menopause.

Erectile dysfunction: In a study, 47 precent of men reported improvement.

Fertility in men: Punicalagin may increase sperm quality and motility (see Health Spotlight).

Hardening of the arteries: Polyphenols appear to reduce plaque formation in the arteries and may help repair blood vessel damage.

High blood pressure: Polyphenols help prevent hardening of the arteries, which can lead to high blood pressure.

Immunity: Vitamin B_6 aids in immune system function and in antibody production; vitamin C boosts the immune system's ability to fight ear infections, colds, and flu.

Lung cancer: Consuming pomegranates may reduce the growth and spread of lung cancer cells.

Prostate cancer: Pomegranate juice shows promise in slowing the growth of cancer and increasing the death of cancer cells.

Skin aging: Copper and antioxidants including vitamin C improve skin health by boosting collagen production.

Skin cancer: Topical creams containing pomegranate have been shown to reduce risk of tumors.

Stroke: Polyphenols may prevent high blood pressure and hardening of the arteries, which reduce risk of stroke.

Wound healing: Phenolic compounds speed healing time.

POMEGRANATE NUTRITION INFORMATION

Serving Size 1 pomegranate, whole

Amount Per Serving

Calories 105	Calories from fat 4
	% Daily Value*
Total Fat 0 grams	0%
Saturated fat 0 gm	0%
Trans fat 0 gm	†
Cholesterol 0 milligrams	0%
Sodium 5 mg	.2%
Total Carbohydrate 26 gm	9%
Dietary fiber 1 gm	4%
Sugars 26 gm	†
Protein 1 gm	2%
Vitamin A	3%
Vitamin C	16%
Calcium	0%
Iron	3%
Also contains:	
Potassium	11%
Vitamin K	9%
Vitamin B_6 (pyridoxine)	8%
Copper	5%
Vitamin E	5%

† Daily Value not established.
* Percent Daily Values are based on a 2,000-calorie diet.

HEALTH SPOTLIGHT

Pomegranate Juice Increases Male Fertility

In a 2008 study, daily consumption of pomegranate juice for seven weeks resulted in increased sperm quality and motility. The study showed decreases in abnormal sperm, increased cell density, and improved motility in rats that drank pomegranate juice compared to those that drank only distilled water. Additionally, the levels of antioxidant enzyme activity in sperm increased in rats that drank pomegranate juice, which researchers surmise contributed to the increased quality of sperm.

QUICK TIPS

❖ The French made grenadine famous. Grenadine is the pomegranate syrup added to Shirley Temples and many cocktails. Unfortunately, most commercial grenadines don't actually contain pomegranate. Make your own by bringing 1 cup pomegranate juice and $3/4$ cup sugar to a boil, reduce the heat and cook at a low boil, stirring occasionally, about 20 minutes or until thickened. Allow the syrup to cool to room temperature. Refrigerate until ready to serve. For a "Shirley Temple" with less sugar, add this syrup to lemon or lime sparkling water and ice.

Pomegranate Dressing

YIELD: $3/4$ CUP

$1/4$ cup pomegranate concentrate*

$1/2$ cup extra virgin olive oil

1 tablespoon Dijon mustard

Black pepper to taste

* Dynamic Health (www.dynamichealth.com) has a lovely, no-sugar-added pomegranate concentrate. The natural tartness makes it a perfect antioxidant-rich substitute for vinegar in salad dressings.

In a small bowl, whisk all the dressing ingredients well. Refrigerate until ready to serve. Use this dressing for the spinach salad recipe on page 190.

* * *

For other recipes and ways of using pomegranate, see: Stuffed Date Appetizer with Pomegranate Dipping Sauce (page 96), Spinach Salad with Whole-Wheat Toast Points (page 191), Strawberry Summer Pudding (page 195).

37. PUMPKIN

Pumpkin has been used as a food and medicine for thousands of years, with evidence of cultivation dating as far back as 5,000 B.C. in Mexico. The Yuma Indians mashed pumpkin seeds and watermelon to make a poultice to treat wounds (the copper in pumpkin seeds may have acted as an antimicrobial). Native Americans also ate strips of pumpkin roasted over an open fire. It is thought that when the Colonists added milk and spices to the empty gourds before roasting, the first "pumpkin pie" was created. This colorful squash is rich in antioxidant carotenoids, including beta-carotene (a precursor of vitamin A), beta-cryptoxanthin, lutein, and zeaxanthin, and is a good source of antioxidant vitamins C and E, known to neutralize free radicals. And pumpkin boasts a whopping 763 percent of the Daily Value of vitamin A per cup! The hearty Pumpkin Potage recipe here is a perfect comfort food on a cold autumn day, and because this soup uses canned pumpkin you can enjoy it year-round. The Pumpkin Pots de Soymilk dessert is a creamy, spicy alternative to pumpkin pie.

HEALTH BENEFITS

Research shows compounds and nutrients found in pumpkin may benefit:

Brain health: Carotenoids can potentially boost brain function and prevent mental decline (see Health Spotlight).

Cataracts: Lutein and zeaxanthin (both found in the eye lens) may slow the development of cataracts.

Heart disease: Eating a diet that includes plenty of carotenoid-rich foods is associated with a lower risk of heart disease.

High blood pressure: Potassium helps lower blood pressure.

Immunity: Carotenoids increase immune function partly by enhancing the function of the immune system's T cells, which help to fight off bacteria, viruses, and other invaders.

Kidney stones: Potassium helps reduce calcium excretion to reduce risk.

Lung cancer: Beta-cryptoxanthin is linked to a lower risk of lung cancer in smokers.

Macular degeneration (age-related): Lutein and zeaxanthin help retain macular pigments in the eye, and antioxidants reduce free-radical damage.

Night blindness: Vitamin A improves nighttime vision by increasing retinol (the most usable form of vitamin A).

Osteoporosis: Potassium increases bone mineral density.

Prostate cancer: Carotenoids appear to support prostate function; a diet high in carotenoid-rich foods is associated with lower risk.

Skin health: Carotenoids increase skin hydration and elasticity.

Stroke: Potassium lowers blood pressure and reduces the stickiness of blood platelets that can cause clots.

PUMPKIN NUTRITION INFORMATION

Serving Size 1 cup canned pumpkin, no salt added

Amount Per Serving

Calories 83 — Calories from fat 6

	% Daily Value*
Total Fat 1 gram	1%
Saturated fat 0 gm	0%
Trans fat 0 gm	†
Cholesterol 0 milligrams	0%
Sodium 12 mg	1%
Total Carbohydrate 20 gm	7%
Dietary fiber 7 gm	28%
Sugars 8 gm	†
Protein 3 gm	6%
Vitamin A	763%
Vitamin C	17%
Calcium	6%
Iron	19%
Also contains:	
Potassium	14%
Magnesium	14%
Vitamin E	12%
Copper	12%

† Daily Value not established.
* Percent Daily Values are based on a 2,000-calorie diet.

HEALTH SPOTLIGHT

Beta-carotene May Prevent Mental Decline

A long-term study of men who supplemented their diets with beta-carotene, found in high amounts in pumpkin, showed less of a decline in cognitive functioning than those who did not, reports the *Archives of Internal Medicine*. Men whose diets included beta-carotene supplements over an eighteen-year period scored significantly higher on cognitive tests including memory exams, which could indicate decreased risk for dementia.

QUICK TIPS

❖ Make sure to purchase "solid-pack" pumpkin with no added ingredients (not pumpkin pie filling).

❖ For pumpkin ice cream: mix $1/2$ cup solid-pack pumpkin, $1/3$ cup packed brown sugar, and a dash of cinnamon with a pint of softened vanilla ice cream. Return to container and refreeze.

❖ Solid-pack pumpkin can be used in place of oil in prepackaged muffin and bread mixes.

Pumpkin Two Ways

As pumpkin is my favorite fruit, I think it works equally well as a starter and as a dessert. So here is an appetizer soup and a sweet custard treat. —ANDI

Pumpkin Potage

YIELD: 8 CUPS

2 stalks lemongrass

$1/2$ cup peanut oil

$1/2$ cup minced shallots

2 tablespoons minced ginger

1 tablespoon minced garlic

2 tablespoons Thai red curry paste

$13/4$ cups homemade or canned vegetable broth

$1/4$ cup Thai fish sauce

$1/4$ cup fresh squeezed lime juice

$1/4$ cup sucanat

13.5 ounces canned coconut milk

29 ounces canned pumpkin

1 tablespoon finely grated lime zest
(zest lime before juicing)

1 cup loosely packed fresh basil leaves,
coarsely chopped

Remove and discard the green portion of the lemongrass stalks. Thinly slice the white portions of the stalks. In a 4-quart stockpot, over low heat warm the oil. Sauté the lemongrass until it is fragrant, about 5 to 7 minutes. Stop if lemongrass starts to take on color. Strain the oil. Discard the lemongrass and return the oil to the stockpot.

Over low heat, sweat the shallots in the infused oil, stirring often, approximately 3 minutes. Add the ginger and garlic. Sweat about 2 more minutes. Stir in the curry paste. Add the vegetable stock, fish sauce, lime juice, and sucanat. Stir well to dissolve the sucanat. Add the coconut milk and pumpkin. Increase the heat to medium and bring the mixture just to a boil stirring constantly. Stir in the lime zest and fresh basil.

Pumpkin Pots de Soymilk

YIELD: 6 RAMEKINS

3 cups soymilk

1 vanilla bean, split lengthwise, scraped,
and cut into large pieces

4 eggs

2 teaspoons sweet curry powder
(our favorite is Penzeys Sweet Curry Powder)

1 teaspoon cinnamon

1 cup canned pumpkin

1 cup maple syrup

Pinch of salt

Preheat oven to 325°F.

In a small saucepan, combine the soymilk, vanilla bean, and scraped seeds. Bring the milk to a simmer. Remove from the heat and allow the mixture to steep about 15 minutes. Strain to remove large vanilla bean pieces.

In a medium bowl, whisk together the eggs, curry powder, cinnamon, pumpkin, maple syrup, and salt. While whisking, slowly pour the warm soymilk mixture into the egg mixture.

Divide the egg and soymilk mixture among six 8-ounce ramekins.

TO CREATE A WATER BATH: Set the ramekins inside a large roasting pan. Place the roasting pan into the oven. Pour warm water into the roasting pan to come three-quarters of the way up the sides of the ramekins. Bake at 325°F for 40 minutes. A knife inserted into the center of the pots de soymilk should come out moist but not have any egg bits clinging to it.

* * *

For other recipes and ways of using pumpkin, see: Pumpkin Oatmeal (page 137).

38. QUINOA

You may be hesitant to cook with it if you can't even pronounce it, but trust us, quinoa (*keen-wah*) deserves a space on your shelves. This whole-grain alternative (actually a protein-rich, gluten-free seed related to spinach and chard) was once a staple of the Inca Indians, who considered it a sacred food and called it "the mother seed." They must have known that it is one of the most complete foods in nature, providing an array of amino acids and enzymes, plant sterols and stanols, along with polyunsaturated fats such as omega-3 fatty acids. This makes it especially ideal for vegetarians and vegans. Quinoa is also packed with phytonutrients, lignans, fiber, and minerals, plus it offers antioxidant protection. Quinoa is so versatile it can be used in soups, salads, and even desserts. In fact, it may be best to eat quinoa as part of a dessert—eating quinoa in the evening may even help you sleep, as it contains tryptophan.

HEALTH BENEFITS

Research shows compounds and nutrients found in quinoa may benefit:

Asthma: Eating a diet that includes plenty of whole grains was found to cut the risk of childhood asthma by 50 percent.

Breast cancer: Eating a diet high in fiber-containing foods is associated with a reduced risk of breast cancer.

Carpal tunnel syndrome: Vitamin B_6 may help alleviate swelling and numbness in the hands and wrists.

Depression: Tryptophan is necessary for the synthesis of the feel-good chemical serotonin; vitamin B_6 helps to convert tryptophan to serotonin.

Diverticulitus: Magnesium, which helps muscles relax, together with fiber, which helps move food through the intestines, can relieve constipation, lowering risk.

Eczema and dermatitis: Eating foods high in manganese is associated with lower incidences of these skin conditions.

Fatigue: Iron and vitamin B$_6$ protect against anemia.

Gallstones: Insoluble fiber speeds the transit time of food through the intestines while reducing bile acid secretion (which can lead to gallstones).

Heart arrhythmias: Magnesium helps keep heart rhythm steady and lowers arrhythmia risk.

Heart disease: Lignans and fiber reduce cholesterol by binding bile and blood cholesterol together and helping to shuttle it out of the body.

High blood pressure: Magnesium lowers blood pressure by helping the blood vessels relax and expand; low levels of magnesium are associated with increased risk.

High cholesterol: Stanols and sterols compete with cholesterol and keep it from being absorbed into the bloodstream.

Insomnia: Tryptophan is a precursor for serotonin, a neurotransmitter that regulates sleep.

QUINOA NUTRITION INFORMATION

Serving Size 1 cup quinoa, cooked

Amount Per Serving

Calories 222	Calories from fat 32
	% Daily Value*
Total Fat 4 grams	5%
Saturated fat 0 gm	0%
Trans fat 0 gm	†
Cholesterol 0 milligrams	0%
Sodium 13 mg	1%
Total Carbohydrate 39 gm	13%
Dietary fiber 5 gm	21%
Sugars 0 gm	†
Protein 8 gm	16%
Vitamin A	0%
Vitamin C	0%
Calcium	3%
Iron	15%
Also contains:	
Manganese	58%
Magnesium	30%
Phosphorus	19%
Copper	18%
Vitamin B$_6$ (pyridoxine)	11%

† Daily Value not established.
* Percent Daily Values are based on a 2,000-calorie diet.

Leg cramps: Magnesium helps to alleviate pregnancy-related leg cramps.

Longevity: Manganese and copper are cofactors in the production of superoxide dismutase (SOD), a powerful antioxidant enzyme that protects against the formation of free radicals that promote aging and disease.

Migraine headache: Magnesium relaxes muscles and nerves and is often low in migraine sufferers.

PMS symptoms: Magnesium helps relieve cramps, irritability, and mood swings.

Type 2 diabetes: Magnesium acts as a cofactor for an enzyme involved in insulin production.

Varicose veins: Copper helps promote blood vessel flexibility.

Wound healing: Lysine encourages tissue growth and repair.

HEALTH SPOTLIGHT

Migraine Headache Help

Quinoa is rich in magnesium, a mineral shown to alleviate migraine headaches. In a study, forty people who had headaches (thirty-six of whom suffered from migraines) were given 1 milligram of intravenous magnesium. Thirty-two of the subjects (80 percent) had complete elimination of headache pain in just fifteen minutes. Relief lasted a few hours for fourteen of the thirty-two subjects, while eighteen experienced relief a full twenty-four hours or more. Of those who experienced longer relief, most had lower magnesium levels before the start of the study. Low magnesium levels have been linked to migraines, while increased intake of magnesium has been associated with fewer migraines.

QUICK TIPS

❖ Sauté zucchini and onion in olive oil and toss into cooked quinoa—for more flavor, when cooking quinoa, substitute chicken or vegetable broth for water.

❖ For an A.M. oatmeal alternative or a P.M. dessert, cook quinoa in soymilk instead of water and add cinnamon and agave or honey.

Quinoa-Chicken Salad

Vinaigrette

$1/4$ cup balsamic vinegar

1 tablespoon Dijon mustard

$1/2$ cup pitted Kalamata olives

$1/2$ cup olive oil

2 garlic cloves, crushed

Salad

1 cup quinoa

2 cups water

$1/2$ cup tightly packed fresh parsley leaves, chopped

1 cup tightly packed fresh basil leaves, chopped

$1/2$ cup diced red onion

$1/2$ cup pitted Kalamata olives, coarsely chopped

$1/2$ cup sundried tomato halves packed in oil,
coarsely chopped

4 ounces fresh mozzarella pearls*

6 cups mixed field greens (such as baby lettuces,
endive, arugula, mache, and frisée)

Chicken

1 pound boneless, skinless, chicken tenders

3 tablespoons vegetable oil

Salt and pepper

* If mozzarella pearls are not available, you can buy a larger piece of fresh mozzarella and cut it into a small dice.

TO MAKE THE VINAIGRETTE: Combine the vinegar, mustard, olives, oil, and garlic in a blender and process until smooth. Refrigerate until ready to use.

TO MAKE THE SALAD: In a 2-quart saucepan, bring the water to a boil. Add the quinoa. Cover and cook over low heat for 12 to 15 minutes until all the water is absorbed. Fluff with a fork and allow the quinoa to cool in the refrigerator while you prepare the rest of the salad. In a large bowl, combine the cooled quinoa with all the other salad ingredients except the field greens.

TO MAKE THE CHICKEN: Season the chicken tenders on both sides with the salt and pepper. Heat the vegetable oil in a large skillet. In the hot oil, brown the chicken on both sides.

TO ASSEMBLE FOR SERVING: Place $1^1/_2$ cups of the field greens on each plate. Top each plate of greens with one-quarter of the quinoa mixture. Lay one-quarter of the warm chicken on top of each plate of quinoa and dress with the vinaigrette.

*   *   *

For other recipes and ways of using quinoa, see: Broccoli Quick Tips (page 60), Cherry-Aki Salmon with Cherry-Studded Quinoa (page 72).

39. RED WINE

"Wine from long habit has become an indispensable for my health . . . I double the doctor's recommendation of a glass and a half of wine a day and even treble it with a friend."
—THOMAS JEFFERSON (1743–1826)

Even before scientific experiments began to prove it, cultures throughout history have praised wine for its health and healing properties. Pliny the Elder, a Roman officer living in the first century A.D. declared, "In wine there is health." Greek doctors prescribed wine for a variety of ailments. Today, red wine is thought to be one of the reasons the Mediterranean diet is so beneficial to the heart. Flavonoids, procyanidins, antioxidants, and primarily resveratrol are among the compounds in red wine thought to be responsible for its health benefits. It has also been found to be a strong antibacterial and antimicrobial that may even help kill bacteria that cause sore throat. The red wine sorbet recipe here made from a shiraz contains no alcohol (it is cooked away). However, the resveratrol content is not affected, as resveratrol molecules are not heat sensitive.

HEALTH BENEFITS

Research shows compounds found in red wine may benefit:

Alzheimer's disease: Resveratrol shows promise in inhibiting formation of Alzheimer's disease plaques.

Asthma: Resveratrol exhibits anti-inflammatory activity in airway epithelial cells.

Blood clots: Resveratrol may inhibit blood clot formation; alcohol may reduce blood clots.

Breast cancer: Resveratrol may help prevent breast cancer by helping balance estrogen.

Cataracts: Research shows resveratrol delays the formation of cataracts.

Cavities: Flavonoids in red wine prevent bacteria from causing tooth decay.

Cholesterol: Resveratrol appears to elevate levels of HDL (good) cholesterol.

Digestive health: Flavonoids in wine help the stomach digest meat.

Heart health: Antioxidants and flavonoids protect blood vessels; resveratrol improves cardiovascular function and prevents artery damage.

Liver health: Resveratrol may reduce liver damage from alcohol.

Longevity: Studies suggest resveratrol could extend life span.

RED WINE NUTRITION INFORMATION

Serving Size 5 ounces of red wine

Amount Per Serving

Calories 100		Calories from fat 0
		% Daily Value*
Total Fat 0 grams		0%
Saturated fat 0 gm		0%
Trans fat 0 gm		†
Cholesterol 0 milligrams		0%
Sodium 7.09 mg		.29%
Total Carbohydrate 2.41 gm		.8%
Dietary fiber 0 gm		0%
Sugars 0 gm		†
Protein .28 gm		.5%
Vitamin A		0%
Vitamin C		0%
Calcium		0%
Iron		0%

† Daily Value not established.

* Percent Daily Values are based on a 2,000-calorie diet.

Obesity: Resveratrol has been found to reduce the number of fat cells in the body; this may help explain the French Paradox, or why the French remain slim despite a high-fat diet—they also drink a lot of wine!

Osteo- and rheumatoid arthritis: With curcumin, resveratrol has been found to reduce inflammation, which could have implications for inflammatory conditions such as arthritis; turmeric (featured on page 210) contains curcumin.

Osteoporosis: Resveratrol may improve bone density.

Prostate cancer: Decreased risk was reported in red wine drinkers (see Health Spotlight).

Type 2 diabetes: Resveratrol helps regulate glucose levels by improving insulin sensitivity.

Prostate Cancer

In a study involving men ages forty to sixty-four who drank red wine, those who drank four to seven glasses of red wine a week over the course of eight years were 52 percent less likely to develop prostate cancer. White wine did not show significant benefits. Drinking beer actually increased the risk of developing prostate cancer. It is speculated that the flavonoids and resveratrol in red wine are responsible for the benefits seen in the study.

QUICK TIP

❖ While it is generally believed that one to two glasses of red wine a day can be healthful, you can obtain the health benefits of resveratrol without the alcohol by cooking with wine. Try adding dry red wine to marinara sauce (homemade or jarred), or to meatballs for a richer flavor. It can be used in place of beef stock in some recipes.

Red Wine and Nectarine Sorbet

YIELD: ABOUT 1 QUART

1 bottle (750 ml) dry red wine such as shiraz

4 chai tea bags

$1/2$ cup light brown sugar or sucanat

2 teaspoons vanilla extract

$1/8$ teaspoon salt

$13/4$ pounds very ripe fresh nectarines (with skins), pitted and sliced

In a 3-quart saucepan, over very low heat, reduce the red wine for an hour. The wine should never come to a boil. There should only be visible steam coming from the top of the liquid. With only 5 minutes left in the hour, add the chai to the warm wine. Allow it to steep for the remainder of the hour. Strain wine and discard tea.

Return the wine to the saucepan. Add the sugar, vanilla, salt, and fruit. Cook for another 10 minutes over low heat. Cool slightly.

Transfer the mixture to the bowl of a food processor. Process it on high until you have completely liquefied the mixture. Pour the mixture through a sieve into a heat-safe bowl. Use a rubber scraper to force as much of the mixture through the sieve as possible. Discard any fibrous bits that remain in the sieve. Put the mixture into the refrigerator and allow it to cool completely. Freeze the mixture in an ice cream maker according to manufacturer's directions. Transfer it to an airtight container and freeze 4 hours before serving.

40. SALMON

It's hard to beat salmon when it comes to healthy oils and nutrition. It's great grilled, added to salads, and tossed in pasta. Cold-water fish like salmon are high in essential omega-3 fatty acids, offering strong protection against heart disease and cancer. Moreover, salmon is packed with vitamins and minerals, which along with omega-3s boost brain power, assisting in cognitive function. There is even research to support its use in helping to mitigate behavior problems including temper tantrums and hyperactivity. Per serving, wild Alaskan salmon provides 105 percent of vitamin B_{12} and 103 percent of selenium. Just one serving of Chinook salmon provides 103 percent of vitamin D (the "sunshine vitamin," linked to cancer protection). And canned salmon is an especially good source of calcium.

HEALTH BENEFITS

Research shows compounds and nutrients found in salmon may benefit:

Alzheimer's disease: Omega-3s appear to slow the accumulation of amyloid beta plaque that results in brain-cell death; niacin-rich diets were found to help lower Alzheimer's risk by 70 percent.

Asthma: Omega-3s help reduce inflammation and increase airflow; diets high in omega-3-containing fish are associated with a 50 percent reduction in childhood asthma; asthma sufferers also tend to have low selenium levels, and salmon is a rich source.

Bipolar disorder: Eating a diet rich in seafood may be effective in reducing risk of bipolar disorder.

Cancer: Selenium and vitamin D have both been shown to be cancer protective; diets that include fish and foods rich in omega-3s are associated with lower risk of a wide variety of cancers.

Cognitive function: Cognitive decline is linked to low levels of docosahexaenoic acid (DHA) and eicosapentaenoic acid (EPA), two types of omega-3 fatty acids.

Colon cancer: Diets high in omega-3s have been shown to lower risk by 37 percent.

Dementia: Research shows a link between higher DHA levels and a reduced risk of dementia.

Depression: Omega-3s may be effective in lifting depression and boosting mood.

Dry eye syndrome: Omega-3s may help reduce risk of dry eye syndrome.

Fertility in men: Vitamin B_{12} may benefit low sperm count.

Heart arrhythmia: Omega-3s protect against abnormal heart rhythms.

Heart attack: Higher omega-3 intake in the diet is linked to a reduced risk of heart attack.

Heart health: Omega-3s are anti-inflammatory and can help protect arteries; vitamin B_{12} inhibits the formation of homocysteine (a potentially toxic chemical and significant risk factor for heart disease).

SALMON NUTRITION INFORMATION

Serving Size $1/2$ fillet (about 7 ounces) wild Atlantic salmon

Amount Per Serving

Calories 281	Calories from fat 113
	% Daily Value*
Total Fat 13 grams	19%
Saturated fat 2 gm	10%
Trans fat 0 gm	†
Cholesterol 109 milligrams	36%
Sodium 87 mg	4%
Total Carbohydrate 0 gm	0%
Dietary fiber 0 gm	0%
Sugars 0 gm	†
Protein 39 gm	78%
Vitamin A	2%
Vitamin C	0%
Calcium	2%
Iron	9%

Also contains:

Vitamin B_{12} (cobalamin)	105%
Selenium	103%
Vitamin B_3 (niacin)	78%
Vitamin B_2 (riboflavin)	44%
Phosphorus	40%
Vitamin B_5 (pantothenic acid)	33%
Vitamin B_1 (thiamine)	30%
Potassium	28%
Copper	25%
Omega-3 fatty acids 3,996 mg	†

Chinook salmon (4 ounces) contains tryptophan (103%) and vitamin D (103%).

† Daily Value not established.

* Percent Daily Values are based on a 2,000-calorie diet.

High blood pressure: Diets high in omega-3s appear to lower blood pressure; potassium lowers high blood pressure.

High cholesterol: Omega-3s and niacin help to lower cholesterol.

High triglycerides: Two servings of fish a week has been shown to lower triglycerides.

Hostile behavior and other behavior problems: In one study, a significant link was found between intake of omega-3s and reductions in hostility.

Hyperactivity: Children taking omega-3s have shown significant improvement in symptoms of ADHD.

Immunity: Vitamin D helps fight infections.

Insomnia: Tryptophan is a precursor for serotonin, a neurotransmitter that regulates sleep.

Leukemia: Eating a diet that includes plenty of fatty fish like salmon could cut the risk of leukemia by 28 percent.

Macular degeneration (age-related): Consuming omega-3-containing fish three times a week may reduce risk by 75 percent.

Obesity: EPA stimulates the secretion of leptin, a hormone that helps regulate food intake.

Osteo- and rheumatoid arthritis: Omega-3s help reduce inflammation and may relieve joint pain.

Osteoporosis: Calcium helps keep bones strong; potassium boosts bone mineral density.

Prostate cancer: Vitamin D is linked to reduced risk; eating salmon just once a week has been associated with a 43 percent lower risk.

Stroke: Eating omega-3-containing fish two to four times per week may drop the risk of ischemic stroke by 18 percent.

Sunburn: Omega-3 fish oils are associated with less DNA damage to skin, which may also benefit skin cancer.

HEALTH SPOTLIGHT

Lower Triglycerides with DHA

Too many triglycerides in the blood has been linked to cardiovascular disease. Statin drugs are widely prescribed to lower triglycerides and cholesterol. However, research shows that docosahexaenoic acid (DHA), an omega-3 fatty acid found in salmon, can effectively lower triglycerides in patients with coronary artery disease (CAD). The study looked at 116 patients with CAD and triglyceride levels of 200 mg/dL or higher. Patients received either 1,000 mg of DHA, or 1,252 mg of DHA and eicosapentaenoic acid (EPA), another omega-3 fatty acid, for eight weeks. Both groups lowered their triglycerides—an average of 21.8 percent in the DHA group, and 18.3 percent in the DHA and EPA group. Researchers say the difference between the groups is not significant, although it is worth noting that DHA can work independently to lower triglyceride levels. The American Heart Association recommends 1,000 mg of EPA/DHA daily for cardio protection.

QUICK TIPS

❖ Choose wild salmon rather than farm raised. Farm-raised salmon carries up to sixteen times greater amounts of polychlorinated biphenyls (PCBs), a carcinogenic compound stored in the fat of the fish that is linked to cancer.

❖ Salmon and fennel (page 100) taste great together.

Smoked Salmon Pasta

YIELD: 4 SERVINGS

1 pound pearl onions

2 tablespoons grape seed oil to sauté, and extra for roasting

1 pint cherry tomatoes

8 ounces cremini mushrooms, thinly sliced

$1/4$ cup chardonnay (or other dry white wine)

3 cloves garlic, finely minced

1 teaspoon orange zest

1 cup evaporated milk

8 ounces smoked salmon, cut into very small pieces

8 ounces whole-wheat penne

Parmesan cheese for garnish

Preheat oven to 350°F.

Blanch the onions in boiling water for 3 minutes. Run them under cold water. Peel the skins. On a baking sheet, toss the onions in just enough grape seed oil to coat. Roast them for one hour. Meanwhile, on another sheet pan, toss the cherry tomatoes in just enough oil to coat. When the onions have been roasting for 30 minutes, put the tomatoes on another rack in the same oven and continue to roast both for the remainder of the hour.

While the vegetables are roasting, sauté the mushrooms in a skillet over low heat just until they are tender, and give up their juices. Add the chardonnay, garlic, and zest. Continue to cook the vegetables over medium heat until the chardonnay is almost evaporated. The mushrooms should just look moist. Add the evaporated milk and continue to cook until the sauce thickens slightly. By this time the onions should be a nice golden brown. Add the onions and the salmon to the sauce. Cook the pasta according to the package directions. Drain the pasta and return it to the warm pot. Pour the mushroom sauce over the warm pasta. Lightly toss in the roasted tomatoes. Garnish with the Parmesan cheese. Serve immediately.

* * *

For other recipes and ways of using salmon, see: Cherry-Aki Salmon with Cherry-Studded Quinoa (page 72), Fennel Quick Tips (100), Turmeric Quick Tips (212).

41. SESAME SEEDS

According to Assyrian legend, the gods drank sesame wine the night before they were inspired to create the Earth. In fact, the use of sesame seeds dates back thousands of years. Egyptians added sesame seeds to bread dough, and Greek warriors carried the seeds with them as a kind of ancient trail mix. It's no wonder—packed with protein and high in minerals such as magnesium, zinc, and calcium, these tiny seeds are nutritional powerhouses. They have long been a part of Asian cooking, as well as Middle Eastern cuisine (tahini, made from ground sesame seeds, is commonly added to hummus). Recently, it has been discovered that sesame seeds contain lignan fibers called sesamin and sesamolin, which lower cholesterol and prevent high blood pressure. Additionally, sesame seeds are a source of phytosterols (plant sterols), which also lower cholesterol, making sesame seeds an especially heart-healthy food. The phytic acid in sesame seeds can lower blood sugar. And a range of minerals in sesame seeds support bone health and could benefit osteoporosis. Tahini sauce is an excellent way to get more of the benefits of sesame seeds in your diet—try this one on the Black Bean Falafel on page 51.

HEALTH BENEFITS

Research shows compounds and nutrients found in sesame seeds may benefit:

Alzheimer's disease: Taking thiamine resulted in improved Alzheimer's disease assessment scale scores.

Anxiety: Low levels of thiamine are associated with anxiety.

Asthma: Magnesium helps prevent airway spasms.

Blood pressure: Magnesium promotes normal blood pressure.

Cancer: Phytosterols have been found to decrease the risk of some cancers.

Colon cancer: Studies show calcium can protect the colon from carcinogens; phytic acid inhibits cancer.

Depression: Thiamine boosted mood in college students in one study; low levels of vitamin B_6 are linked to depression.

Digestive health: Fiber improves digestion and is linked to a reduced risk of hemorrhoids and diverticulitis (bulging tissue pouches in the colon); thiamine is important for hydrochloric acid production (which is necessary for proper digestion).

Fatigue: Iron combats anemia that can lead to fatigue and low energy; thiamine has been shown to reduce symptoms of post-workout fatigue.

High blood pressure: Sesamolin helps prevent high blood pressure.

High cholesterol: Phytosterols and sesamolin may lower cholesterol (see Health Spotlight).

Immunity: Zinc stimulates immune-cell activity, even a mild deficiency can impair immune function and increase susceptibility to infections; phytosterols strengthen the immune system.

Liver health: Sesamin protects the liver from oxidative damage.

SESAME SEEDS NUTRITION INFORMATION	
Serving Size 1 ounce whole sesame seeds, toasted	
Amount Per Serving	
Calories 158	Calories from fat 112
	% Daily Value*
Total Fat 13 grams	21%
Saturated fat 2 gm	9%
Trans fat 0 gm	†
Cholesterol 0 milligrams	0%
Sodium 3 mg	.125%
Total Carbohydrate 7 gm	2%
Dietary fiber 4 gm	16%
Sugars 0 gm	†
Protein 5 gm	10%
Vitamin A	0%
Vitamin C	0%
Calcium	28%
Iron	23%
Also contains:	
Copper	35%
Manganese	35%
Magnesium	25%
Phosphorus	18%
Vitamin B_1 (thiamine)	15%
Zinc	13%
Vitamin B_6 (pyridoxine)	11%

† Daily Value not established.
* Percent Daily Values are based on a 2,000-calorie diet.

Migraine headache: Magnesium relaxes muscles and nerves and is often low in migraine sufferers; calcium helps prevent migraines.

Osteoporosis: Calcium, magnesium, manganese, phosphorus, and zinc are all needed to make healthy bone; calcium, along with manganese and zinc, also helps slow bone loss.

PMS symptoms: Calcium and magnesium help relieve symptoms including headache, bloating, and moodiness.

Reaction time: Taking thiamine resulted in increased reaction times.

Rheumatoid arthritis: Copper activates anti-inflammatory enzymes that help reduce arthritis-related pain; it also aids in forming collagen and elastin.

Sleep problems: Magnesium has been shown to relieve sleep problems associated with menopause.

Type 2 diabetes: Phytic acid lowers blood sugar.

Varicose veins: Copper helps promote blood vessel flexibility; vitamin B_6 is often recommended for varicose veins to prevent lesions in blood vessels and reduce appearance of varicose veins.

HEALTH SPOTLIGHT

Lower Cholesterol with Sesame Seeds

A 2005 study published in the *Journal of Agricultural and Food Chemistry* tested twenty-seven different nut and seed products for phytosterol content. It was discovered that sesame seeds and wheat germ contained the highest concentration of phytosterols (more than 400 milligrams per 100 grams). Phytosterols work to lower cholesterol by blocking cholesterol absorption in the intestines. Phytosterols also work to boost the immune system.

QUICK TIPS

❖ Use tahini dressing on salads or as a veggie dip.

❖ Toast sesame seeds in a skillet for about 4 minutes or in a 350°F oven for 10 to 15 minutes until lightly browned, and sprinkle on steamed or roasted veggies.

Tahini Sauce

YIELD: 2 CUPS OF SAUCE

$1/_2$ cup tahini paste

$1/_4$ cup fresh squeezed lime juice

$3/_4$ cup unsweetened soymilk

$1/_4$ cup extra virgin olive oil

3 garlic cloves, crushed

$1/_2$ cup packed fresh cilantro

$1/_4$ teaspoon smoked paprika

$1/_2$ teaspoon salt

Combine all of the ingredients in the bowl of a food processor. Process on high until mixture is a smooth paste. Serve as a sauce over falafel, as a salad dressing, or as a dip with pita chips.

42. SHIITAKE MUSHROOMS

They have been used in Chinese medicine for 6,000 years and are a symbol of longevity, said to revitalize "chi" or vital energy. Commonly added to miso soup, shiitake mushrooms contain high amounts of a powerful antioxidant called ergothioneine, in addition to a compound called lentinan that has been found to fight cancer as well as viruses including the flu. Another component of shiitake mushrooms called eritadenine lowers cholesterol, and pepsin and trypsin aid in digestion. Shiitake mushrooms have been used through the centuries for such conditions, as well as for arthritis, headaches and fatigue (today, it's often used as an alternative treatment for chronic fatigue syndrome). Additionally, one cup of shiitake mushrooms contains 65 percent of the Daily Value of copper, which helps the body produce melanin necessary for skin, eye, and hair color. Some people take copper to help reverse gray hair.

HEALTH BENEFITS

Research shows compounds and nutrients found in shiitake mushrooms may benefit:

Acne: Zinc helps prevent acne and regulate the activity of oil glands, and is often low in acne sufferers.

Cancer: Lentinan has been shown to destroy cancer cells.

Cavities: Lentinan may reduce plaque formation.

Common cold and flu: Lentinan helps bolster immune defenses.

Depression: Low levels of B-complex vitamins are linked to depression; B vitamins are necessary for the synthesis of the feel-good chemical serotonin that helps regulate anxiety and mood.

Digestive health: Pepsin and trypsin help the stomach digest protein.

Healthy hair and skin color: Copper helps the body produce melanin, the pigment responsible for hair and skin color.

Hepatitis B: Lentinan has demonstrated effectiveness in protecting against hepatitis B.

High cholesterol: Research shows eritadenine lowers levels of LDL (bad) cholesterol; niacin helps increase levels of HDL (good) cholesterol and improve circulation.

Immunity: Lentinan helps promote an increase in T-cell activity (see Health Spotlight).

Longevity: Mushrooms including shiitake contain high amounts of ergothioneine, a powerful antioxidant that helps protect against the formation of free radicals, which promote aging and disease.

Macular degeneration (age-related): Shiitake promotes production of interferon, a protein that helps prevent blood vessel overgrowth; zinc reduces vision loss; selenium may reduce risk.

Thyroid health: Selenium plays a key role in thyroid hormone metabolism.

Varicose veins: Copper promotes blood vessel flexibility.

SHIITAKE MUSHROOMS NUTRITION INFORMATION

Serving Size 1 cup shiitake mushrooms, cooked

Amount Per Serving

Calories 81	Calories from fat 3

	% Daily Value*
Total Fat 0 grams	0%
Saturated fat 0 gm	0%
Trans fat 0 gm	†
Cholesterol 0 milligrams	0%
Sodium 6 mg	.25%
Total Carbohydrate 21 gm	7%
Dietary fiber 3 gm	12%
Sugars 5 gm	†
Protein 2 gm	4%
Vitamin A	0%
Vitamin C	1%
Calcium	0%
Iron	4%

Also contains:

Copper	65%
Vitamin B_5 (pantothenic acid)	52%
Selenium	51%
Vitamin B_2 (riboflavin)	51%
Zinc	15%
Vitamin B_6 (pyridoxine)	12%
Vitamin B_3 (niacin)	11%

† Daily Value not established.
* Percent Daily Values are based on a 2,000-calorie diet.

HEALTH SPOTLIGHT

Shiitake Mushrooms Boost Immunity

Shiitake has been shown to power up the immune system against bacterial and viral infections—even HIV. The compound lentinan appears to be responsible for these positive effects. In one study, lentinan (given with a standard drug) was shown to help patients with HIV infection maintain higher CD4 cell counts, or T-cell count, for a longer period of time than those who received the drug alone.

QUICK TIPS

❖ Add fresh skiitake mushrooms to miso soup (page 132), omelets, or kabobs.

❖ For a tea—especially if you have a cold or the flu—simmer a few dried shiitake mushrooms in water for about 15 minutes, strain, and drink.

Shiitake Mushroom Tilapia

YIELD: SERVES 6

2 tablespoons olive oil

4 garlic cloves, minced

2 shallots, minced

1 pound shiitake mushrooms, sliced

1 cup chardonnay or other dry white wine

3 plum tomatoes, diced

1 tablespoon fresh minced tarragon

6 fillets (about 4 to 6 ounces each) of tilapia

Salt and pepper to taste

$1/2$ cup half and half

In a large skillet over medium heat, sauté the garlic and shallots just until fragrant. Add the mushrooms and chardonnay. Turn the heat to medium-high. Cook, stirring often, until almost all of the chardonnay has evaporated. Add the tomatoes and tarragon. Stir to combine. At this point, you can hold the sauce until the fish is done cooking. Season the fish with salt and pepper and pan fry fillets about 4 minutes on each side. To finish the sauce, add the half and half and cook, stirring until slightly thickened. Serve the mushroom sauce over the fish fillets.

*   *   *

For other recipes and ways of using shiitake mushrooms, see: Millet Hash (page 129), Miso Quick Tips (page 132), Stir-Fried Eggplant in Miso Sauce (page 132).

43. SPINACH

Popeye swallowed a can of spinach anytime he needed a little extra strength. And although you may not develop bulging muscles immediately like Popeye, new research shows that eating spinach may indeed stimulate muscle growth, due in part to the action of a natural steroid called phytoecdysteroids. Of course, the high iron content of spinach also helps boost energy and strength. And spinach is even higher in vitamin K—one cup of the cooked leaves contains about 1,000 percent of this nutrient, important for bone and heart health. This leafy green is proving to be an extremely powerful cancer fighter as well, with an array of nutrients, and phytochemicals and flavonoids that have demonstrated anti-cancer activity. Eating spinach may even help your skin form a kind of natural "sunscreen"!

HEALTH BENEFITS

Research shows compounds and nutrients found in spinach may benefit:

Alzheimer's disease: Folate with vitamin B_{12} (not present in spinach) was shown to improve Alzheimer's symptoms.

Cancer (breast, prostate, ovarian, and pancreatic cancers): Phytonutrient flavonoids including kaempferol, and carotenoids including lycopene reduce risk (see Health Spotlight).

Cataracts: Lutein and zeaxanthin (both found in the eye lens) may help slow the development of cataracts.

Cognitive decline: Antioxidants prevent damage from free radicals, and may increase the brain's ability to send signals and retain function of motor skills and learning capacity.

Colorectal cancer: Studies show vitamins C and E, beta-carotene, and folate can prevent mutations in colon cells.

Depression: Kaempferol acts as an antidepressant.

Fatigue: Iron combats anemia that can lead to fatigue and low energy.

Heart attack: Folate, which lowered heart attack risk by 55 percent in one study, inhibits the formation of homocysteine (a potentially toxic chemical and significant risk factor for heart disease).

Heart disease: Diets low in magnesium are associated with a higher risk of heart disease.

Liver cancer: Research shows chlorophyllin, derived from chlorophyll found in leafy greens, is effective in fighting liver cancer.

Macular degeneration (age-related): Lutein, along with vitamins A, C, and E, helps slow age-related macular degeneration.

Muscle development: Phytoecdysteroids may increase development of muscles by up to 20 percent.

Osteo- and rheumatoid arthritis: Beta-carotene and vitamin C are anti-inflammatory.

Osteoporosis: Vitamin K helps improve bone density, in part, by slowing calcium loss in bone; iron may promote osteoblast activity (cells that build bone).

Skin cancer: Flavonoids and other phytonutrients have been shown to boost natural sun protection factor (SPF) in skin.

Stroke: Folate inhibits the formation of homocysteine (a potentially toxic chemical and significant risk factor for blood vessel damage).

SPINACH NUTRITION INFORMATION

Serving Size 1 cup spinach, raw

Amount Per Serving

Calories 7 — Calories from fat 0

	% Daily Value*
Total Fat 0 grams	0%
Saturated fat 0 gm	0%
Trans fat 0 gm	†
Cholesterol 0 milligrams	0%
Sodium 24 mg	0%
Total Carbohydrate 1 gm	.33%
Dietary fiber 1 gm	4%
Sugars 0 gm	†
Protein 1 gm	2%
Vitamin A	56%
Vitamin C	14%
Calcium	3%
Iron	5%
Also contains:	
Vitamin K	181%
Folate	15%
Manganese	13%
Magnesium	6%
Potassium	5%
Vitamin E	3%

† Daily Value not established.
* Percent Daily Values are based on a 2,000-calorie diet.

HEALTH SPOTLIGHT

Reduced Risk of Ovarian Cancer

An eighteen-year study involving more than 65,000 women examined flavonoid intake of their diets, including the flavonoid called kaempferol, which is found in large amounts in spinach. The study revealed that women who ate foods rich in kaempferol (including spinach, broccoli, and tea) reduced their risk of ovarian cancer by 40 percent.

QUICK TIPS

❖ A large bunch of fresh spinach cooks down quickly in a skillet with a little olive oil and garlic for a quick, healthy side dish.

❖ Sautéed spinach is fantastic in an omelet with feta cheese.

Spinach Salad with Whole-Wheat Toast Points

YIELD: 2 DINNER-SIZE SALADS

Toast Points

4 slices whole-wheat bread

2 tablespoons olive oil

Salad

Water

1 to 2 tablespoons white vinegar

6 cups fresh, clean baby spinach

$1/4$ of a small red onion, thinly sliced

$1/2$ cup walnuts, toasted (see directions on page 112)

2 ounces prosciutto, sliced into $1/4$-inch strips

$1/2$ cup pomegranate seeds

2 tablespoons Parmesan cheese, freshly grated

2 whole eggs for poaching

TO MAKE TOAST POINTS: Preheat oven to 350°F. Trim only the outermost crust from each slice of bread. You should be left with neat rectangles. Cut across the diagonal of each of the rectangles creating 2 triangles. Place the triangles on a baking sheet and brush the tops with a light coat of olive oil. Bake for 5 to 7 minutes, until they just start to turn golden. Remove them to a cooling rack while you prepare the salad.

TO MAKE THE SALAD: In a small shallow saucepan, bring about 2 inches of water and 1 tablespoon of the white vinegar to a simmer. Crack one egg into a small prep bowl. With the water still at a simmer, gently slide the egg into the water. Maintain the simmer and allow the entire white of the egg to cook. The yolk should still be liquid. This takes about 4 minutes. Use a slotted spoon to remove the egg. Allow the egg to drain on paper towels until you are ready to plate the salad. Repeat this process with the second egg.

Divide the spinach evenly between two dinner plates. Top with sliced red onion, toasted walnuts, sliced prosciutto, pomegranate seeds, and grated cheese. Put four toast points around the edges of the plate for garnish. Top each salad with a warm poached egg and the pomegranate dressing (page 159). Serve immediately.

* * *

For other recipes and ways of using spinach, see: Avocado Quick Tips (page 37).

44. STRAWBERRIES

These heart-shaped berries have long been considered a food fit for lovers, whether chocolate-dipped or served with champagne. It is said that in medieval times, strawberry soup was served to newly married couples at their wedding reception. But aside from stirring feelings of love and passion, strawberries are good for the heart in other ways, too, with antioxidants including an abundance of vitamin C, along with phenols and flavonoids, and even omega-3 fatty acids. The red color comes from anthocyanins, powerful cell-protecting antioxidants. And a phenol called ellagitannin found in strawberries guards against cancer. The list goes on. Take a look.

HEALTH BENEFITS

Research shows compounds and nutrients found in strawberries may benefit:

Asthma: Phenols and vitamin C have anti-inflammatory effects in lungs.

Cancer (liver and prostate cancers): Ellagitannin, omega-3 fatty acids, and anthocyanins and other flavonoids have been shown to slow tumor growth.

Common cold: Vitamin C boosts immunity and may reduce cold symptoms.

Dementia: Research shows vitamin C improves circulation and protects against free-radical damage; omega-3s have been associated with enhanced cognitive function.

Gingivitis: Vitamin C promotes healing, especially of bleeding gums.

Heart health: Phenols protect against free-radical damage to the heart muscle; omega-3s help protect heart muscle cells and control blood clotting.

High blood pressure: Potassium lowers blood pressure.

High cholesterol: Phytosterols lower cholesterol by blocking its absorption in the intestines; fiber lowers cholesterol by binding bile with cholesterol and helping to shuttle it out of the body.

Irritable bowel syndrome: Soluble fiber may relieve symptoms including gas, pain, and bloating.

Macular degeneration (age-related): Eating three or more servings of fruit a day has been found to lower risk of macular degeneration.

Muscle soreness: Vitamin C has been shown to reduce delayed-onset muscle soreness post-workout.

Osteo- and rheumatoid arthritis: Phenols act as anti-inflammatories; vitamin C has been shown to protect against inflammatory arthritis involving two or more joints, as well as reduce free-radical damage and inflammation.

Osteoporosis: Manganese is important for bone health and retaining bone.

PMS symptoms: Manganese and magnesium may reduce irritability.

Pregnancy: Folate protects against a number of congenital malformations, including neural tube birth defects.

Skin health: Vitamin C aids in collagen formation and protects against free-radical damage.

STRAWBERRIES NUTRITION INFORMATION	
Serving Size 1 cup strawberries, fresh	
Amount Per Serving	
Calories 49	Calories from fat 4
	% Daily Value*
Total Fat 0 grams	0%
Saturated fat 0 gm	0%
Trans fat 0 gm	†
Cholesterol 0 milligrams	0%
Sodium 2 mg	.08%
Total Carbohydrate 12 gm	4%
Dietary fiber 3 gm	12%
Sugars 7 gm	†
Protein 1 gm	2%
Vitamin A	0%
Vitamin C	149%
Calcium	2%
Iron	3%
Also contains:	
Manganese	29%
Folate	9%
Potassium	7%
Magnesium	5%
Copper	4%
Omega-3 fatty acids 38.8 mg	†
† Daily Value not established.	
* Percent Daily Values are based on a 2,000-calorie diet.	

Stroke: Potassium, magnesium, and omega-3s work together to reduce risk by lowering blood pressure, reducing cholesterol, preventing blood clots, and keeping blood vessels flexible.

Weight loss and weight control: Fiber-containing foods provide a feeling of fullness; fiber slows digestion, helping to keep blood sugar levels stable and reduce insulin spikes that can trigger cravings and encourage fat storage.

HEALTH SPOTLIGHT

Arthritis Pain? Try Strawberries

Phenols in strawberries are anti-inflammatory, acting in the same way in the body to reduce pain as anti-inflammatory drugs such as aspirin and ibuprofen. The phenols in strawberries reduce the activity of the cyclooxygenase (COX) enzyme, just like the COX-inhibitor drugs do. Too much of this enzyme leads to inflammation, which contributes to both rheumatoid and osteoarthritis, as well as other inflammatory-related conditions. And besides tasting better than swallowing a pill, strawberries will give you none of the unwanted side effects of drugs.

QUICK TIPS

❖ The best way to welcome summer? Fresh strawberries and real whipped cream!

❖ Try sliced strawberries in green salads, along with walnuts and gorgonzola cheese.

❖ Pick frozen strawberries over dried—phenols and vitamin C remain intact in frozen strawberries. Dried strawberries lose their vitamin C.

❖ Buy organic—strawberries don't have much of a natural protective covering. (You'll also get more antioxidants from organic fruit.)

Strawberry Summer Pudding

YIELD: 8 SERVINGS

$1/4$ cup cold water

1 ($1/4$ ounce) envelope gelatin

1 commercially made or homemade
angel food cake that serves 8

$3/4$ cup thawed 100% berry juice concentrate*

$11/4$ cups tawny port

15 to 18 large basil leaves, torn into 2 to 3 pieces each

1 teaspoon vanilla extract

Pinch salt

1 pound fresh strawberries,
hulled and quartered

Special Equipment

Plastic wrap

Bowl, 6-cup volume

Small plate that fits within the top rim of the 6-cup bowl

*We use the pomegranate-cherry juice concentrate available in the freezer section of most supermarkets. Our favorite brand is Old Orchard.

In a small bowl, bloom the gelatin in the cold water for at least 10 minutes. Set aside for later use.

Line a 6-cup volume bowl with plastic wrap. Cut the angel food cake into quarters then slice each quarter into about 6 thin slices. Line the bottom and sides of the 6-cup bowl with slightly overlapping pieces of the angel food cake. Save about a third of the slices for the top of the pudding.

In a medium saucepan, bring the juice concentrate, tawny port, basil leaves, vanilla extract, and salt to a boil. Once at a rolling boil, reduce heat to low and simmer for 7 minutes. Strain out and discard the basil leaves and return the juice/port mixture to the pan. Add the strawberries to the pan. Bring the mixture back to a boil. Reduce the heat to low and simmer about 3 minutes, until the strawberries start to become soft. Remove from the heat and immediately stir in the bloomed gelatin. Stir until the gelatin has completely dissolved. Pour the strawberries and all of the juice/port mixture into the cake-lined bowl. Use the remaining pieces of cake to cover the strawberries. Loosely lay a piece of plastic wrap over the top of the pudding. Place a small plate, preferably one that fits within the top rim of bowl, on top of the plastic wrap. Use large cans to weigh down the plate and compress the pudding. Refrigerate overnight.

When you are ready to serve, remove the small plate and plastic wrap from the top of the bowl. Invert a large serving platter over the top of the pudding bowl. Turn the bowl and platter over. The pudding will release from the bowl onto the platter. Peel away the layer of plastic that was used to line the bowl. Serve in slices. It can be served with whipped cream.

45. SWEET POTATOES

Sweet potatoes may have been one of the first things man cooked when he discovered fire. There is evidence that people have been eating sweet potatoes since prehistoric times, as far back as 10,000 years ago. Sweet potatoes hail from Central America, but spread throughout the world after Christopher Columbus brought back sweet potatoes to Europe from his first voyage. There are about 400 different varieties of the sweet potato, including white, pink, and purple varieties. The most common is the yellow-orange variety, which is particularly high in vitamin A, while purple varieties contain high amounts of anthocyanins, giving them even more potent antioxidant power. Overall, sweet potatoes are an excellent source of vitamins A and C, antioxidants that destroy free radicals that can damage cells and lead to heart problems and cancer. Sweet potatoes also contain unique root proteins that act as antioxidants. The skin of the sweet potato is three times higher in antioxidants than that of the potato itself; however, if you eat the skin, be sure to choose organic sweet potatoes.

HEALTH BENEFITS

Research shows compounds and nutrients found in sweet potatoes may benefit:

Asthma: Antioxidants help to fight inflammation and increase airflow.

Atherosclerosis: Vitamins A and C block early free-radical damage that can lead to thickening and hardening of the arteries.

Brain health: Beta-carotene may protect brain cells from oxidative damage, helping to reduce cognitive decline.

Cancer (lung, skin, breast, and prostate cancers): Eating a diet that includes plenty of carotenoids has been shown to cut the risk of cancer.

Cataracts: Vitamin A is necessary for proper eye function and protection from free radicals.

Depression: Low levels of B-complex vitamins are linked to depression; B vitamins are necessary for the synthesis of the feel-good chemical serotonin that helps regulate anxiety and mood.

Diverticulitis: Fiber helps promote healthy digestion, prevent constipation, and lower risk.

Emphysema: Vitamin A shows promise in treatment.

Heart attack: Eating carotenoid-rich foods including carrots and squash daily may reduce risk of heart attack by 60 percent; vitamin B_6 helps reduce dangerous homocysteine levels, a risk factor for atherosclerosis.

High cholesterol: Fiber reduces cholesterol by binding bile with cholesterol and helping to shuttle it out of the body.

Night blindness: Vitamin A with zinc was shown in a study to improve night vision.

SWEET POTATOES NUTRITION INFORMATION	
Serving Size, 1 large sweet potato, baked in skin	
Amount Per Serving	
Calories 162	Calories from fat 2
	% Daily Value*
Total Fat 0 grams	0%
Saturated fat 0 gm	0%
Trans fat 0 gm	†
Cholesterol 0 milligrams	0%
Sodium 65 mg	3%
Total Carbohydrate 37 gm	12%
Dietary fiber 6 gm	24%
Sugars 12 gm	†
Protein 4 gm	8%
Vitamin A	692%
Vitamin C	59%
Calcium	7%
Iron	7%
Also contains:	
Manganese	45%
Vitamin B_6 (pyridoxine)	26%
Magnesium	12%
Vitamin B_2 (riboflavin)	11%
† Daily Value not established.	
* Percent Daily Values are based on a 2,000-calorie diet.	

Osteo- and rheumatoid arthritis: Antioxidants act as anti-inflammatories to alleviate swelling and pain.

PMS symptoms: Manganese may help with mood swings.

Skin health: Beta-carotene acts as a natural sunscreen (see Health Spotlight).

Stroke: Vitamin B_6 helps reduce harmful homocysteine levels, a risk factor for atherosclerosis as well as stroke.

Type 2 diabetes: Carotenoids have been shown to have a positive effect on insulin resistance.

HEALTH SPOTLIGHT

Natural Sunscreen

Exposure to ultraviolet A (UVA) rays from sunlight can speed aging of the skin by increasing oxidative stress. Now, researchers have found that beta-carotene (found in large amounts in sweet potatoes) may offer some protection. Using human skin cells, the study showed beta-carotene suppresses enzymes activated by UVA light, which lead to degradation of the extracellular matrix of the skin. In addition, the scientists found that UVA rapidly destroys beta-carotene in the cells, a sign that beta-carotene has to be replenished after exposure to sunlight. Beta-carotene supplementation has been reported to have a mild sunscreen effect.

QUICK TIP

❖ To make sweet potato fries, cut sweet potatoes into french-fry-sized strips or even easier—use pre-cut sweet potato strips. Toss in a bowl with olive oil and arrange in a single layer in a shallow baking pan. Sprinkle with salt and ground black pepper. Bake the fries at 350°F for about 20 minutes or until the edges are slightly browned.

Smoky Sweet Potatoes

Potato Filling

2 pounds fresh sweet potatoes

6 ounces cream cheese, at room temperature

$1/2$ cup Greek-style yogurt

$1/4$ cup 100% pure maple syrup

2 eggs

$1/2$ teaspoon ground cinnamon

2 to 4 teaspoons minced chipotle in adobo sauce
(depending on your tolerance for heat)

$1/2$ teaspoon salt

Topping

$3/4$ cup sliced almonds

3 tablespoons 100% pure maple syrup

$1/2$ teaspoon adobo sauce from the chipotle chili container

$1/8$ teaspoon salt

TO PREPARE THE POTATOES: Preheat oven to 350°F. Bake the sweet potatoes for 45 to 70 minutes, until fork tender. The cooking time will vary depending on how large your sweet potatoes are. Meanwhile, prepare the rest of the recipe.

TO PREPARE THE TOPPING: Combine all the topping ingredients in a small bowl and set aside for later use.

In the bowl of a stand mixer, beat the cream cheese on high to soften. With the beater running, add the yogurt, maple syrup, eggs, cinnamon, chipotle, and salt. Beat until smooth. Reserve until the sweet potatoes are baked and are cool enough to handle.

Peel the warm sweet potatoes and dice them into large pieces. In the work bowl of a food processor, process the diced sweet potatoes until you have a smooth paste.

With the processor running, add the cream cheese mixture and process until completely combined. Transfer the mixture to a 1-quart soufflé dish. Sprinkle the almond topping evenly over the sweet potato mixture. Bake at 350°F for 30 to 40 minutes. Just the edges should start to take on some color. The center will jiggle if shaken but should not be liquid.

46. TOMATOES

Italy was the first to embrace the tomato as a food outside of South America, where tomatoes were eaten by the Aztecs as long ago as 500 B.C. They have since become the cornerstone of the Mediterranean diet. From plum (Roma) to heirloom and even the fried green variety, tomatoes are one of the most popular "fruits" in the world. Red tomatoes contain lycopene, which has shown promise in some studies to protect against prostate and other cancers, and are a good source of chromium. Although the Food and Drug Administration (FDA) has denied requests from tomato-product companies to include claims on their packaging that lycopene benefits cancer, research remains promising, according to Dr. Edward Giovannucci of the Harvard School of Public Health. Some evidence suggests it may be the whole tomato (lycopene along with other compounds that work synergistically—not just lycopene alone) that is responsible for cancer protection. In addition, tomatoes have an array of nutrients important for heart health.

HEALTH BENEFITS

Research shows compounds and nutrients found in tomatoes may benefit:

Asthma: Antioxidants help ease inflammation and increase airflow.

Cancer (prostate, breast, endometrial, lung, and colorectal cancers): Lycopene appears to protect cells from oxidants.

Cataracts: Vitamin A is necessary for proper eye function and protection from free radicals; vitamin A intake is associated with a 39 percent reduced risk of development.

Colon cancer: Folate has been linked to cancer protection and reduced risk.

Fertility: Antioxidants and lycopene are linked to enhanced fertility.

Heart disease: Lycopene, folate, and vitamin B_6 help metabolize dangerous homocysteine levels, a risk factor for atherosclerosis.

High blood pressure: Potassium lowers blood pressure.

High cholesterol: Niacin helps to lower cholesterol and improve circulation.

Immunity: Vitamin C enhances the immune system's ability to fight infections.

Macular degeneration (age-related): Carotenoids with vitamins A and C work to protect eyes from free-radical damage and vision loss.

Osteo- and rheumatoid arthritis: Vitamin C acts as an anti-inflammatory to alleviate swelling and pain.

Osteoporosis: Vitamin K helps improve bone density, in part, by slowing calcium loss in bone.

Skin protection: Vitamin A acts as a mild sunscreen.

Stroke: Vitamin C and potassium reduce risk of stroke.

Type 2 diabetes: Chromium helps regulate glucose levels by improving insulin sensitivity.

TOMATOES NUTRITION INFORMATION

Serving Size 1 medium tomato

Amount Per Serving

Calories 22	Calories from fat 2
	% Daily Value*
Total Fat 0 grams	0%
Saturated fat 0 gm	0%
Trans fat 0 gm	†
Cholesterol 0 milligrams	0%
Sodium 6 mg	.25%
Total Carbohydrate 5 gm	2%
Dietary fiber 1 gm	6%
Sugars 3 gm	†
Protein 1 gm	2%
Vitamin A	20%
Vitamin C	26%
Calcium	1%
Iron	2%
Also contains:	
Vitamin K	12%
Potassium	8%
Chromium	7.5%
Manganese	7%
Folate	5%
Niacin	5%
Vitamin B$_6$ (pyridoxine)	5%
Omega-3 fatty acids 3.7 mg	†

† Daily Value not established.
* Percent Daily Values are based on a 2,000-calorie diet.

HEALTH SPOTLIGHT

Women Should Eat More Tomatoes

According to a study from Harvard Medical School, lycopene, an antioxidant in tomatoes, reduces the risk of heart disease in women. The study analyzed blood samples of nearly 500 women who developed cardiovascular disease, and 500 women who had not developed the disease. They found that women with the highest levels of lycopene in the blood had a 33 percent lower risk of developing cardiovascular disease. Other studies have found that lycopene is associated with reduced cardiovascular disease risk in men as well. Lycopene can be found watermelon and pink grapefruit in addition to tomatoes.

QUICK TIPS

❖ Lycopene is more available to the body if tomatoes are cooked. For easy broiled tomatoes, arrange sliced plum or beefsteak tomatoes on a baking sheet. Drizzle with olive oil, and sprinkle with salt and freshly ground black pepper. Top with fresh basil and/or Parmesan cheese if desired. Broil about 5 minutes.

❖ Small heirloom tomatoes with balsalmic dressing make a great snack or side, or add color to a green salad.

Tomato-Seafood Chowder

YIELD: APPROXIMATELY 3 QUARTS

$1/4$ to $1/2$ cup olive oil

1 small brown onion, diced small

1 medium carrot, diced small

1 small fennel bulb, diced small

2 ribs celery, diced small

1 small bell pepper, diced small

4 large cloves garlic, smashed

$1/2$ cup parsley leaves, coarsely chopped

8 ounces cremini mushrooms, sliced

2 cups chardonnay or other dry white wine

1 28-ounce can tomato puree

1 28-ounce can diced tomatoes

1 cup tomato juice

2 cups bottled clam juice

$1/4$ cup fresh squeezed lemon juice

12 ounces red potato, diced into medium chunks

2 6.5-ounce cans clams in juice

1 2-ounce can anchovies, drained and smashed
with the back of a fork

15 to 20 large, fresh basil leaves, coarsely chopped

2 sprigs of fresh oregano, leaves only finely minced

1 8-inch rosemary sprig, leaves only, finely minced

$1/2$ pound cooked baby bay shrimp

Salt to taste

In a large stockpot, over a low flame, heat about $1/4$ cup of the olive oil. Add the onions and cook, stirring infrequently, just until they start to take on some color. Add the carrot, fennel, celery, bell pepper, garlic, parsley, and mushrooms. Add more oil as needed. Continue to cook, stirring infrequently until all vegetables are soft, about 15 minutes. Add the wine. Simmer to reduce the liquid by about half, approximately 10 minutes. Stir in the tomato puree, diced tomatoes, tomato juice, clam juice, lemon juice, potatoes, canned clams with their juice, and smashed anchovies. Simmer over low heat for 1 hour. Stir often. The total volume should be reduced by about a quarter. Stir in the basil, oregano, and rosemary. Simmer on low another 10 minutes. Add the shrimp. Season with salt to desired taste and serve immediately.

*   *   *

For other recipes and ways of using tomatoes, see: Anchovy Quick Tips (page 14), Anchovy-Avocado Appetizer (page 15), Apricot Moroccan-Style Stew (page 23), Arugula Brunch Stack (page 27), Avocado Quick Tips (page 37), Avocado-Tuna Wraps (page 37), Black Bean Falafel (page 51), Coffee-Braised Pork Loin (page 82), Fennel Quick Tips (page 100), Tapenade (page 141), Quinoa-Chicken Salad (page 169), Smoked Salmon Pasta (page 179), Shiitake Mushroom Tilapia (page 187).

47. TUNA

Tuna is not only an excellent source of protein but also of omega-3 fatty acids, essential fats that cannot be made by the body. Typically, the modern processed diet contains many more omega-6 fatty acids, found in commonly used oils such as corn and safflower oils. This can lead to an unhealthy imbalance of omega-3 and omega-6 fats in the body, which promotes inflammation and diseases related to inflammation such as heart disease and arthritis. The omega-3 fats docosahexaenoic acid (DHA) and eicosapentaenoic acid (EPA) found in tuna can help prevent or correct an imbalance. Omega-3s are absorbed by cell membranes and positively affect the way cells respond, even aiding in destroying cancer cells. In addition to providing omega-3s in the diet, tuna offers benefits from nutrients including selenium, phosphorus, magnesium, and vitamin B_{12}.

HEALTH BENEFITS

Research shows compounds and nutrients found in tuna may benefit:

Alzheimer's disease: Vitamin B_{12} has been shown to improve Alzheimer's symptoms and is often low in people with the disease.

Anxiety: Magnesium helps reduce anxiety by having a calming effect.

Asthma: Omega-3s help reduce inflammation and increase airflow; diets high in omega-3-containing fish are associated with a 50 percent reduction in childhood asthma; asthma sufferers also tend to have low selenium levels, and tuna is a rich source.

Atherosclerosis: Twice-weekly fish consumption is associated with reduced risk.

Bipolar disorder: Eating a diet rich in seafood may be effective in reducing risk of bipolar disorder.

Breast cancer: Cancer cell growth dropped by 25 percent when treated with DHA and EPA.

Colon cancer: Diets rich in EPA and DHA were found to lower risk by 37 percent.

Deep vein thrombosis (including blood clots in veins that cause swelling and pain): Eating fish high in omega-3s once a week may lower risk.

Depression: Inflammation caused by consuming too many omega-6 fats in relation to omega-3s may decrease serotonin levels, which influence mood.

Eczema: Taking DHA supplements over eight weeks improved symptoms significantly.

Fatigue: Vitamin B_{12} has been shown to fight chronic fatigue syndrome and increase energy.

Heart arrhythmia: Canned tuna and other broiled or baked fish are associated with a 28 percent lower risk.

Heart attack: Daily servings of omega-3-rich fish like tuna lowered coronary heart disease risk by 42 percent.

TUNA NUTRITION INFORMATION		
Serving Size 3 ounces bluefin tuna		
Amount Per Serving		
Calories 122	Calories from fat 38	
		% Daily Value*
Total Fat 4 grams		6%
Saturated fat 1 gm		5%
Trans fat 0 gm		†
Cholesterol 32 milligrams		11%
Sodium 33 mg		1%
Total Carbohydrate 0 gm		0%
Dietary fiber 20 gm		6%
Sugars 0 gm		†
Protein 1 gm		2%
Vitamin A		37%
Vitamin C		0%
Calcium		1%
Iron		5%
Also contains:		
Vitamin B_{12} (cobalamin)		134%
Selenium		44%
Phosphorus		22%
Vitamin B_1 (thiamine)		14%
Magnesium		11%
Omega-3 fatty acids 1,103 mg		†

† Daily Value not established.

* Percent Daily Values are based on a 2,000-calorie diet.

High blood pressure: Increased consumption of omega-3s has been associated with lower blood pressure.

High triglycerides: Two servings of fish a week has been shown to lower triglycerides.

Hostility: A statistically significant difference in "hostility scores" was found between adolescents who ate omega-3-rich fish compared to those who did not.

Inflammation: Resolvin, a lipid made from EPA, eases inflammation in the body, lessening the need for anti-inflammatory drugs.

Kidney cancer: A fifteen-year study showed a 44 percent lower risk with consumption of fatty fish such as tuna at least once a week.

Liver detoxification: Selenium helps break down toxins and aids in detoxification.

Macular degeneration (age-related): Omega-3s, especially from tuna, have shown significant protection to the eyes.

Obesity: EPA stimulates the secretion of leptin, a hormone that helps regulate food intake.

Osteoporosis: Phosphorus and calcium work together to form bone.

Prostate cancer: Selenium is needed for proper prostate function; risk has been shown to be lower in men with higher selenium levels.

Restless leg syndrome: This common condition may be linked to a vitamin B_{12} deficiency.

Rheumatoid arthritis: Consuming tuna was found to reduce the need for NSAIDs.

Stroke: Eating fish such as tuna, even one to three times a month, showed reduced risk.

Sunburn: Omega-3s are associated with less DNA damage to skin, which may also benefit skin cancer.

Type 2 diabetes: Increased consumption of fish improves insulin response.

HEALTH SPOTLIGHT

No More Dry Eye

If you suffer from dry eye syndrome (DES), adding tuna to your diet can help. In a study of about 40,000 women ranging in age from forty-five to eighty-four, those who ate the most tuna (five to six servings per week) had a 68 percent lower risk of DES. Women who ate two to four servings of tuna per week had a 19 percent lower risk of DES. Overall, findings showed that women who consumed the highest amounts of omega-3 fatty acids had a 17 percent lower risk of dry eye syndrome compared with those who consumed the least. Conversely, a diet high in omega-6 fats, but low in omega-3s, increased DES risk significantly.

QUICK TIP

❖ Canned tuna is a good source of omega-3 fats, too, providing about 239 milligrams per 3 ounces (comparable to that found in 3 ounces of fresh yellowfin). But buy water-packed tuna. The added oils in oil-packed tuna may replace some of the natural omega-3s, leaving you with about 172 milligrams of omega-3s per 3 ounces.

Tuna Tartare Appetizer Salad

YIELD: 4 APPETIZER-SIZE SALADS

1 tablespoon mirin

1 tablespoon soy sauce

1 teaspoon rice vinegar

$1/2$ teaspoon finely grated fresh ginger

1 teaspoon toasted sesame oil

8 ounces sushi grade tuna, diced small

1 scallion, green and white parts, thinly sliced

$1^1/2$ teaspoons wasabi paste

2 tablespoons safflower or canola mayonnaise

1 cup avocado, diced small

2 cups mixed field greens
(baby lettuces, endive, arugula, mache, and frisée)

In a medium bowl, whisk well to combine the mirin, soy sauce, rice vinegar, grated ginger, and sesame oil. Gently toss in the tuna and scallions. Mix to insure that all tuna is evenly covered with dressing. This can be made up to an hour before needed. Refrigerate until needed.

In a small bowl, combine the wasabi paste and the mayonnaise. Gently fold in the diced avocado just enough to coat it with the dressing.

To plate for serving, put ¹/₄ cup of field greens on a small plate. Top the greens with a quarter of the avocado mixture. Top the avocado with a quarter of the tuna mixture. Serve immediately.

*   *   *

For other recipes and ways of using tuna, see: Avocado-Tuna Wraps (page 37).

48. TURMERIC

Although this Indian spice has been revered in Ayurvedic medicine for millennia, Western medicine is only now beginning to understand its mysterious healing powers. For centuries, turmeric (found in curry powder) has been used to treat conditions including gas, toothache, menstrual cramps, and bruising. In Chinese medicine, it is prescribed for depression. More recently, studies show that curcumin (an antioxidant and the main biologically active compound in turmeric) can dissolve Alzheimer's disease plaques and fight cancer. It has antiviral, antifungal, and antibacterial properties, which may help explain its effectiveness against ulcers and viral infections, and is a source of vitamin B_6. Turmeric is widely available in capsule form, but we think this Macadamia-Pineapple Curry recipe is a better way to take your turmeric.

HEALTH BENEFITS

Research shows compounds and nutrients found in turmeric may benefit:

Allergies: Studies show curcumin reduces allergic response.

Alzheimer's disease: Curcumin protects brain cells from oxidative damage and is thought to boost immune-cell activity that helps clear amyloid beta plaque in the brain (see Health Spotlight).

Anemia: Turmeric contains 16 percent of the Daily Value of iron in just 1 tablespoon; iron is essential for oxygenation of the blood and energy production.

Breast cancer: Curcumin appears to inhibit a protein that causes tumor growth.

Childhood leukemia: Curcumin may mitigate effects of environmental pollutants and inhibit leukemia cell formation.

Colon cancer: Curcumin was found to decrease formation of pre-cancerous polyps in the lower intestine.

Cystic fibrosis: Curcumin corrected the formation of a mutated protein responsible for the disease in one study.

Fat metabolism: Curcumin benefits the liver by improving fat metabolism.

Gallstones: Populations with a turmeric-rich diet develop fewer gallstones.

Heart disease: Vitamin B_6 inhibits the formation of homocysteine (a potentially toxic chemical and significant risk factor for heart disease).

Heartburn: Curcumin can relieve symptoms, but overuse may cause stomach upset.

High cholesterol: Curcumin was found to increase production of proteins that create LDL (bad) cholesterol receptors, which help clear more LDL from the body.

TURMERIC NUTRITION INFORMATION	
Serving Size 1 tablespoon turmeric	
Amount Per Serving	
Calories 24	Calories from fat 6
	% Daily Value*
Total Fat 1 gram	1%
Saturated fat 0 gm	1%
Trans fat 0 gm	†
Cholesterol 0 milligrams	0%
Sodium 3 mg	.125%
Total Carbohydrate 4 gm	1%
Dietary fiber 1 gm	6%
Sugars 0 gm	†
Protein 1 gm	2%
Vitamin A	0%
Vitamin C	3%
Calcium	1%
Iron	16%
Also contains:	
Vitamin B_6 (pyridoxine)	6%
Manganese	26%
† Daily Value not established.	
* Percent Daily Values are based on a 2,000-calorie diet.	

Irritable bowel syndrome: Curcumin may benefit symptoms of IBS, possibly by inhibiting an inflammatory agent known as NF-kappa B.

Liver detox: Turmeric appears to induce formation of the liver detoxification enzyme glutathione S-transferase.

Multiple sclerosis: Doses of curcumin equivalent to that found in a typical Indian diet resulted in significant reduction of disease symptoms.

Osteo- and rheumatoid arthritis: Curcumin acts as an anti-inflammatory by inhibiting the COX-2 enzyme that triggers pain-producing substances.

Pain: Curcumin can help relieve pain from inflammatory-related conditions.

Prostate cancer: Turmeric combined with cauliflower reduced prostate cancer cell growth in a study.

Psoriasis: Taking curcumin shows promise in treating psoriasis.

Type 2 diabetes: Studies show curcumin may help control blood sugar levels.

Wound healing: Curcumin prevents oxidative damage to skin cells.

HEALTH SPOTLIGHT

Turmeric Benefits Alzheimer's Disease

It is the bisdemethoxycurcumin, an active ingredient found in turmeric root, that has been shown to increase immune-system activity, helping Alzheimer's patients to clear the amyloid beta plaques associated with the condition. In healthy patients, immune cells called macrophages destroy abnormal cells and pathogens, which clears amyloid beta plaques. In Alzheimer's patients, this process is not effective. Turmeric, however, was found to boost macrophage activity to normal levels, helping to clear the plaques.

QUICK TIP

❖ Mix turmeric with sour cream and use as a veggie dip. Try with sweet potato fries (page 199), or add a dollop to salmon.

Macadamia-Pineapple Curry

YIELD: 6 SERVINGS

6 ounces macadamia nuts

1 15-ounce can coconut milk

3 tablespoons vegetable oil

1 14-ounce package extra-firm tofu,
drained, diced small

2 cups fresh pineapple, diced small

3 large cloves garlic, minced

2 tablespoons finely minced fresh ginger

2 tablespoons yellow curry powder
(our favorite is Penzeys Sweet Curry Powder)

$1/4$ cup fresh squeezed lemon juice

Salt to taste

6 scallions, green and white parts, cut into 1-inch pieces

In a food processor or blender, grind the macadamia nuts until they are powdery. With the machine running, add the coconut milk in a thin stream. Set aside for later use.

In a large skillet heat the vegetable oil. Add the tofu cubes. Cook over medium heat stirring occasionally until the tofu cubes are golden brown on all sides. Add the pineapple, garlic, and ginger. Stir until the garlic and ginger are fragrant. Reduce the heat to low. Add the curry powder and stir until the curry is evenly distributed. Add the coconut milk/ macadamia nut mixture. Cook, stirring frequently, until the sauce begins to thicken. Add the lemon juice. Salt to taste. Stir in the scallions. Serve over rice or noodles.

* * *

For other recipes and ways of using turmeric, see: Black Bean Falafel (page 51).

49. WATERMELON

Watermelons were prized in the hot Egyptian desert for their water content—watermelons are 92 percent water!—and are even depicted on ancient Egyptian hieroglyphics. That other 8 percent is loaded with an amazing array of healthful compounds. Citrulline, which increases the amino acid arginine in the body, helps to relax blood vessels and lower blood pressure. The antioxidant lycopene has been shown to fight prostate and many other cancers. And watermelon is packed with other antioxidants to fight free radicals including vitamin A as beta-carotene, and vitamin C. Recently, vitamin A has been shown to help repair skin damage as a result of too much time in the sun—good thing watermelon is a staple of backyard summer barbeques.

HEALTH BENEFITS

Research shows compounds and nutrients found in watermelon may benefit:

Asthma: Antioxidants reduce inflammation that can restrict airways.

Atherosclerosis: Vitamins A and C help stop the oxidation of cholesterol, protecting against the formation of plaque in the arteries.

Cancer (prostate, breast, endometrial, lung, and colorectal cancers): Lycopene protects cells from oxygen damage and shows promise in fighting these cancers.

Colon cancer: Vitamin C and beta-carotene prevent damage to the lining of the colon.

Erectile dysfunction: Citrulline is involved in the production of nitric oxide, the same compound enhanced by Viagra (see Health Spotlight).

High blood pressure: Citrulline increases arginine production, which converts to nitric oxide that relaxes blood vessels, plus potassium decreases blood pressure.

Immunity: Vitamin C enhances the immune system's ability to fight ear infections, colds, and flu.

Irritable bowel syndrome: Soluble fiber may relieve symptoms including gas, pain, and bloating.

Macular degeneration (age-related): Eating three or more servings of fruit a day may lower risk.

Migraine headache: Magnesium relaxes blood vessels and is associated with lower incidence of migraines.

Muscle soreness: Vitamin C benefits delayed-onset muscle soreness post-workout.

Osteo- and rheumatoid arthritis: Vitamin C reduces inflammation and free-radical damage within joints; it is also essential for production and maintenance of collagen, a major protein found in cartilage that helps cushion joints.

PMS symptoms: Magnesium helps reduce symptoms including headache, bloating, and moodiness.

Skin damage from sun: Vitamin A offers some UV protection and aids in tissue repair and healing.

Stroke: Vitamins A and C and potassium reduce risk of stroke.

Type 2 diabetes: Citrulline helps produce arginine, which has been shown to improve insulin sensitivity.

WATERMELON NUTRITION INFORMATION

Serving Size 1 cup watermelon balls

Amount Per Serving

Calories 46	Calories from fat 2

	% Daily Value*
Total Fat 0 grams	0%
Saturated fat 0 gm	0%
Trans fat 0 gm	†
Cholesterol 0 milligrams	0%
Sodium 2 mg	.08%
Total Carbohydrate 12 gm	4%
Dietary fiber 1 gm	2%
Sugars 10 gm	†
Protein 1 gm	2%
Vitamin A	18%
Vitamin C	21%
Calcium	1%
Iron	2%
Also contains:	
Potassium	5%
Magnesium	4%
Vitamin B$_1$ (thiamine)	3%
Vitamin B$_6$ (pyridoxine)	3%
Copper	3%

† Daily Value not established.
* Percent Daily Values are based on a 2,000-calorie diet.

HEALTH SPOTLIGHT

Watermelon May Benefit Erectile Dysfunction

Nitric oxide production in the body is increased by taking the popular erectile dysfunction drug Viagra. Nitric oxide works by lowering blood pressure and relaxing blood vessels. But by eating watermelon or drinking its juice, a process begins in the body that ultimately leads to increased nitric oxide production as well. Watermelon is high in citrulline, an amino acid our bodies use to make arginine, which, in turn, is used to make nitric oxide. In a study, volunteers drinking three 8-ounce glasses of watermelon juice a day for three weeks had blood levels of arginine that were 11 percent higher than in a control group that did not drink the juice. Volunteers who drank six daily 8-ounce glasses of watermelon juice for three weeks had arginine levels 18 percent higher than in a control group.

QUICK TIPS

❖ Freeze watermelon chunks (remove rinds and seeds) for a cool low-cal treat.

❖ Drizzle agave nectar over watermelon slices.

Watermelon Chiller

YIELD: 2 SERVINGS

2 tablespoons agave syrup
$1/4$ cup unsweetened soymilk
$1/2$ cup Greek-style yogurt
8 ounces seedless watermelon, diced small

Eight hours before serving, freeze the watermelon on a plastic or parchment lined baking sheet.

In the jar of a blender, combine the agave syrup, soymilk, and yogurt. Add the frozen watermelon to the blender a few chunks at a time, allowing each addition to blend completely before adding the next. As more watermelon is incorporated, the beverage will become very thick. Toward the end you may have to stop the blender between additions to stir the mixture with a rubber scraper in order to insure a smooth beverage. This one is healthy enough for breakfast but yummy enough for dessert. Serve immediately.

50. YOGURT

The 1980s wouldn't be the same without it, but the frozen kind doesn't usually contain the beneficial bacteria that make yogurt so good for you. It was soured milk drunk by Bulgarian peasants that led to the discovery of probiotics, the beneficial cultures found in yogurt. In the early 1900s, scientist Elie Metchnikoff observed that the Bulgarians typically lived to a ripe, old age. Metchnikoff became convinced that their health and longevity were linked to microbes in the milk they drank, identified as lactobacilli. He won the Nobel Prize for this discovery. It has since been discovered that such cultures indeed play diverse roles in our health, populating the gut with bacteria necessary for a healthy immune system, digestion, and much more. Yogurt is also high in iodine, calcium, phosphorus, and riboflavin. And even if you're lactose intolerant, you can still enjoy yogurt, as the enzymes in yogurt destroy the lactose. So join the "culture club"!

HEALTH BENEFITS

Studies have shown cultures and nutrients found in yogurt may benefit:

Allergies: Yogurt is linked to reduced inflammation and allergy symptoms (see Health Spotlight).

Arthritis: Research shows the probiotic lactobacillus can reduce inflammation and lessen symptoms.

Bad breath: Yogurt lowers hydrogen sulfide and other compounds that can lead to halitosis.

Bladder cancer: Eating yogurt every day was shown to lower risk.

"Brain fog": Yogurt contains tyrosine, an amino acid that promotes brain health and alertness.

Cataracts: Riboflavin deficiency has been linked to cataracts.

Cholesterol: Regular consumption of yogurt has been found to lower LDL (bad) cholesterol and raise HDL (good) cholesterol.

Colon cancer: Yogurt inhibits colon tumor growth by fighting carcinogens that promote cancer.

Depression: Vitamin B_{12} is associated with more successful outcomes in treatment for depression.

Diarrhea: Yogurt helps replace lost beneficial bacteria and reduce symptoms.

Digestion: Active "live" cultures benefit digestive problems.

Eczema: Probiotics in yogurt reduce risk of eczema.

Gingivitis: Yogurt has been shown to reduce harmful bacteria that can lead to gum disease.

Goiter: Iodine deficiency can lead to this rare condition.

High blood pressure: Potassium lowers blood pressure.

Immunity: Yogurt cultures boost immune function; in one study, the yogurt culture *L. rhamnosus* increased immune activity in the elderly.

Irritable bowel syndrome: Probiotics may alleviate symptoms including gas, pain, and bloating.

YOGURT NUTRITION INFORMATION

Serving Size 1 cup low-fat yogurt, plain

Amount Per Serving

Calories 154	Calories from fat 33

	% Daily Value*
Total Fat 4 grams	6%
Saturated fat 2 gm	12%
Trans fat 0 gm	†
Cholesterol 15 milligrams	5%
Sodium 171 mg	7%
Total Carbohydrate 17 gm	6%
Dietary fiber 0 gm	0%
Sugars 17 gm	†
Protein 13 gm	26%
Vitamin A	2%
Vitamin C	3%
Calcium	45%
Iron	1%
Also contains:	
Iodine	58%
Phosphorus	38%
Vitamin B_2 (riboflavin)	34%
Vitamin B_{12} (cobalamin)	25%
Potassium	18%
Zinc	16%
Selenium	13%
Magnesium	12%

† Daily Value not established.

* Percent Daily Values are based on a 2,000-calorie diet.

Longevity: Yogurt cultures may help extend life span.

Migraine headache: Magnesium relaxes muscles and nerves and has been shown to reduce frequency of attacks.

Osteoporosis: Yogurt contains lactoferrin, a milk protein that appears to stimulate osteoblast activity (cells that build bone); calcium and phosphorus work together to maintain strong bones.

Prostate cancer: Selenium is needed for proper prostate function and has been shown to fight cancer.

Rosacea: Riboflavin has been shown to increase resistance to *Demodex* mites (*Demodex folliculorum*), found in larger numbers on the skin of rosacea sufferers.

Tooth decay: Yogurt has been shown to reduce harmful bacteria contributing to plaque and cavities.

Ulcers: *Lactobacillus acidophilus* and *Bifidobacterium lactis* may suppress *H. pylori* infections known to cause peptic ulcers.

Weight control and weight loss: Calcium may help reduce body fat and retain more lean muscle mass.

Yeast infections: A study found that women who eat yogurt have fewer yeast infections.

HEALTH SPOTLIGHT

Hay Fever Fighter

Allergy sufferers consuming the probiotic *Lactobacillus casei Shirota* (LcS) showed reduced immune response to grass pollen in a study. Volunteers between the ages of eighteen and forty-five took a daily milk drink with or without LcS. According to blood samples, those taking the probiotic had significantly reduced levels of antibodies associated with allergic immune response compared to a control group. At the same time, IgG, a marker indicating protection against allergic reactions, increased in the group taking probiotics.

QUICK TIPS

❖ Look for the words "live, active cultures" when buying yogurt, as well as brands that specify cultures added after pasteurization—heat from pasteurization can destroy healthy bacteria.

❖ Yogurt with added sugars may counteract the positive effects of yogurt cultures—choose plain yogurt and add fresh fruit and alternative sweeteners like agave nectar instead.

Muesli

Muesli is a hearty mixture of yogurt, oats, and a handful of antioxidant-rich ingredients. For a comforting, substantial breakfast make up a batch the night before and it will be ready and waiting for you in the morning.

Muesli Base

YIELD: 1 SERVING

1 cup plain Greek-style yogurt

$^1/_4$ cup rolled oats

Choose one of the following variations. Combine the yogurt, oats, and all the ingredients from your chosen variation. Mix well and store covered, overnight, in the refrigerator.

Almond-Cherry Variation

$^1/_4$ cup dried cherries

2 tablespoons honey

$^1/_2$ teaspoon almond extract

$^1/_4$ cup sliced almonds

Apple-Cinnamon Variation

$^1/_3$ cup dried apples, coarsely chopped

$^1/_2$ teaspoon ground cinnamon

2 tablespoons 100% pure maple syrup

$^1/_4$ cup chopped pecans

Yogurt

Chocolate-Peanut Butter Variation

2 tablespoons chopped dark chocolate (70% or darker)

2 tablespoons agave syrup

2 tablespoons natural, unsweetened peanut butter

Coffee-Coconut Variation

1 teaspoon instant coffee powder

2 tablespoons flax meal

2 tablespoons dried unsweetened coconut

1 tablespoon sucanat

1 teaspoon vanilla extract

Date-Pine Nut Variation

6 dates, chopped

1 tablespoon minced crystallized ginger

1 tablespoon honey

$1/4$ cup pine nuts

Goji-Cardamom Variation

$1/4$ cup goji berries

$1/2$ teaspoon cardamom

2 teaspoons wheat germ

1 tablespoon sucanat

Matcha-Blueberry Variation

1 teaspoon matcha powder

$1/4$ cup dried blueberries

$1/4$ cup chopped macadamia nuts

1 tablespoon sucanat

* * *

For other recipes and ways of using yogurt, see: Almond Quick Tips (page 10), Blueberry Quick Tips (page 55), Blueberry Quick Bread (page 56), Broccoli Lunch Pockets (page 60), Black Bean Burritos with Spicy Chili Salsa (page 77), Cucumber Relish (page 87), Grapefruit Breakfast Napoleon (page 111), Matcha Panna Cotta (page 124), Smoky Sweet Potatoes (page 200), Watermelon Chiller (page 216).

References

All nutrition facts information from nutritiondata.com unless otherwise noted.

Agave Nectar

Puyvelde L. American Society for Microbiology. "In vitro and in vivo activates of a triterpenoid saponin extract (PX-6518) from the plant Maesa balansae against visceral Leishmania species." *Antimicrob Agents Chemother* 2004 Jan; 48: 130–136.

Han LK, Zheng YN, Xu BJ, et al. "Saponins from platycodi radix ameliorate high fat diet-induced obesity in mice." American Society for Nutritional Sciences. *J Nutr* 2002; 132: 2241–2245.

Coxam V. "Inulin-type fructans and bone health: state of the art and perspectives in the management of osteoporosis." *Br J Nutr* 2005; 93(Suppl 1): S111–S123.

Dahl W, Whiting S, Isaac T, et al. "Effects of thickened beverages fortified with inulin on beverage acceptance, gastrointestinal function, and bone resorption in institutionalized adults." *Nutrition* 2005; 21: 308–311.

Daubioul C, Rousseau N, Demeure R, et al. "Dietary fructans, but not cellulose, decrease triglyceride accumulation in the liver of obese Zucker fa/fa rats." *J Nutr* 2002; 132: 967–973.

Glycemic Solutions. "Clinical assessment of glycemic index and load for Blue Agave nectar." (June 2009). Available online at: www.blueagavenectar.com/glycemictestingofagavenectar.html.

Kim YS, Kim JS, Choi SU, et al. "Isolation of a new saponin and cytotoxic effect of saponins from the root of Platycodon grandiflorum on human tumor cell lines." *Planta Med* 2005; 71: 566–568.

Kolida S, Meyer D, Gibson GR. "A double-blind placebo-controlled study to establish the bifidogenic dose of inulin in healthy humans." *EJCN* 2007; 61: 1189–1195.

Quílez, AM, Saenz MT, García R, et al. "Phytochemical analysis and anti-allergic study of *Agave intermixta Trel.* and *Cissus sicyoides L.*" *J Pharmacol* 2004; 56: 1185–1189.

Raschka L, Daniel H. "Mechanisms underlying the effects of inulin-type fructans on calcium absorption in the large intestine of rats." *Bone* 2005; 37: 728–735.

Szilagyi A. "Use of prebiotics for inflammatory bowel disease." *Br J Nutr* 2005; 93 (Suppl 1): S73–S90.

Trautwein EA, Rieckhoff D, Erbersdobler HF. "Dietary inulin lowers plasma cholesterol and triacylglycerol and alters biliary bile acid profile in hamsters." *J Nutr* 1998; 128: 1937–1943.

US Department of Agriculture. "Inulin may help with iron uptake, too." *ScienceDaily.com* 2008 Jan 2008. Available online at: www.sciencedaily.com/?/releases/2008/01/080106133238.htm.

Watzl BN, et al. "Inulin, oligofructose and immunomodulation." *Br J Nutr* 2005; 93 (Suppl 1): S49–S55.

Almonds

Abbey M, Noakes M, Belling GB, et al. "Partial replacement of saturated fatty acids with almonds or walnuts lowers total plasma cholesterol and low-density-lipoprotein cholesterol." *Am J Clin Nutr* 1994; 59: 995–999.

Albert CM, Willet WC, Manson JE, et al. "Nut consumption and the risk of sudden and total cardiac death in the Physicians' Health Study." Abstract. American Heart Association, Nov 9–11, 1998.

Bes-Rastrollo M, Sabate J, Gomez-Gracia E, et al. "Nut consumption and weight gain in a Mediterranean cohort: the SUN study." *Obesity* (Silver Spring) 2007; 15: 107–116.

Blomhoff R, Carlsen MH, Andersen LF, et al. "Health benefits of nuts: potential role of antioxidants." *Br J Nutr* 2008; 99: 447–448.

Calon F, Lim GP, Yang F, et al. "Docosahexaenoic acid protects from dendrite pathology in an Alzheimer's disease mouse model." *Neuron* 2004; 43: 633–645.

Christen WG, Liu S, Glynn RJ, et al. "Dietary carotenoids, vitamins C and E, and risk of cataract in women: a prospective study." *Arch Ophthalmol* 2008; 126: 102–109.

Chung-Yen C, Milbury PE, Lapsley K, et al. "Flavonoids from almond skins are bioavailable and act synergistically with vitamins C and E to enchance hamster and human LDL resistance to oxidation." *J Nutr* 2005; 135: 1366–1373.

Crowley JD, Traynor DA, Weatherburn DC. "Enzymes and proteins containing manganese: an overview." *Met Ions Biol Syst* 2000; 37: 209–278.

Daily Plate, The. "Raw almonds." *Dailyplate.com* 2010. Available online at: www.thedailyplate.com/nutrition-calories/food/365/raw-almonds.

Fraser G, Sabate J, Beeson LW, et al. "A possible effect of nut consumption on risk of coronary heart disease." *Archives of Internal Medicine* 1992; 152: 1416–1424.

Fraser GE. "Nut consumption, lipids, and risk of a coronary event." *Clin Cardiol* 1999; 22 (Suppl 7): S11–S15.

Hu FB, Stampfer MJ. "Nut consumption and risk of coronary heart disease: A review of epidemiologic evidence." *Curr Atheroscler Rep* 1999; 1: 204–209.

Hu FB, Stampfer MJ, Manson JE, et al. "Frequent nut consumption and risk of coronary heart disease in women: prospective cohort study." *BMJ* 1998; 317: 1341–1345.

Jenkins DJ, Kendall CW, Marchie A, et al. "Direct comparison of dietary portfolio vs. statin on C-reactive protein." *Eur J Clin Nutr* 2005 Jul; 59: 851–860.

Josse AR, Kendall CW, Augustin LS, et al. "Almonds and postprandial glycemia—a dose-response study." *Metabolism* 2007 Mar; 56: 400–404.

Kris-Etherton PM, et al. "High-monounsaturated fatty acid diets lower both plasma cholesterol and tria-cylglycerol concentrations." *Am J Clin Nutr* 1999; 70: 1009–1015.

Kris-Etherton PM for the AHA Nutrition Committee. "Monounsaturated fatty acids and risk of cardiovascular disease." *Circulation* 1999; 100: 1253–1258.

Mauskop A, Altura BM. "Role of magnesium in the pathogenesis and treatment of migraines." *Clin Neurosci* 1998; 5(1): 24–27.

Morris MC, et al. "Consumption of fish and n-3 fatty acids and risk of incident Alzheimer disease." *Arch Neurol* 2003; 60: 940–946.

Sacks FM. "Weight reduction: a comparison of a high unsaturated fat diet with nuts versus a low-fat diet." Findings presented at the Experimental Biology Meeting, April 1998.

References

Anchovies

Morris MC, et al. "Consumption of fish and n-3 fatty acids and risk of incident Alzheimer disease." *Arch Neurol* 2003; 60: 940–946.

Powers HJ, Hill MH, Welfare M. "Responses of biomarkers of folate and riboflavin status to folate and riboflavin supplementation in healthy and colorectal polyp patients (The FAB$_2$ Study)." *Cancer Epidemiol Biomarkers Prev* 2007; 16: 2128–2135.

Cell Division. "Omega-3 kills cancer cells." *ScienceDaily.com* 2009 Apr 5. Available online at: www.sciencedaily .com/releases/2009/04/090401200441.htm.

Apples

Olsson ME, Gustavsson KE, Andersson S. "Inhibition of cancer cell proliferation in vitro by fruit and berry extracts and correlations with antioxidant levels." *J Agric Food Chem* 2004 Dec; 52: 7264–7271.

Bazzano LA, He J, Ogden LG, et al. "Dietary fiber intake and reduced risk of coronary heart disease in US men and women: the NHANES I epidemiologic follow-up study." *Arch Intern Med* 2003 Sep 8; 163: 1897–1904.

Boyer J and Liu RH. "Apple phytochemicals and their health benefits." *Nutri J* 2004 May; 3: 5.

Dai Q, Borenstein AR, Wu Y, et al. "Fruit and vegetable juices and Alzheimer's disease: the Kame Project." *Am J Med* 2006 Sep; 119: 751–759.

Davis PA, Polagruto JA, Valacchi G, et al. "Effect of apple extracts on NF-kappaB activation in human umbilical vein endothelial cells." *Exp Biol Med* 2006 May; 231: 594–598.

Eberhardt M, Lee C, Liu RH. "Antioxidant activity of fresh apples." *Nature* 2000; 405: 903–904.

Fernandez ML. "Soluble fiber and nondigestible carbohydrate effects on plasma lipids and cardiovascular risk." *Curr Opin Lipidol* 2001 Feb; 12: 35–40.

Honow R, Laube N, Schneider A, et al. "Influence of grapefruit-, orange- and apple-juice consumption on urinary variables and risk of crystallization." *Br J Nutr* 2003 Aug; 90: 295–300.

Huxley R and Neil H. "The relation between dietary flavonol intake and coronary heart disease mortality: a meta-analysis of prospective cohort studies." *Eur J Clin Nutr* 2003; 57: 904–908.

Kaul TN, Middleton E, Ogra PL. "Antiviral effect of flavonoids on human viruses." *J Med Virol* 1985; 15: 71–79.

Knekt P, Jarvinen R, Reunanen A, et al. "Flavonoid intake and coronary mortality in Finland: a cohort study." *BMJ* 1996 Feb 24; 312: 478–481.

Liu RH, Liu J, Chen B. "Apples prevent mammary tumors in rats." *J Agric Food Chem* 2005; 53: 2341–2343.

Mayo Clinic. "Natural substances in fruits and vegetables may be potential treatment for prostate cancer. *ScienceDaily*.com 2001 Mar 27. Available online at: www.sciencedaily.com/releases/2001/03/010327081312.htm.

Middleton E. "Effect of flavonoids on basophil histamine release and other secretory systems." *Prog Clin Biol Res* 1986; 213: 493–506.

Musci I and Pragai BM. "Inhibition of virus multiplication and alteration of cyclic AMP level in cell cultures by flavonoids." *Experientia* 1985; 41: 930–931.

Ogasawara H and Middleton E. "Effect of selected flavonoids on histamine release (HR) and hydrogen peroxide (H2O2) generation by human leukocytes [abstract]." *J Allergy Clin Immunol* 1985; 75 (Suppl): 184.

Puel C, Quintin A, Mathey J, et al. "Prevention of bone loss by phloridzin, an apple polyphenol, in ovariectomized rats under inflammation conditions." *Calcif Tissue Int* 2005 Nov; 77(5): 311–318.

Sable-Amplis R, Sicart R, Agid R. "Further studies on the cholesterol-lowering effect of apple in humans: biochemical mechanisms involved." *Nutr Res* 1983; 3: 325–328.

Solovchenko A and Schmitz-Eiberger M. "Significance of skin flavonoids for UV-B-protection in apple fruits." *J Exp Bot* 2003 Aug; 54(389): 1977–1984.

Sun J, Chu Y, Wu X, et al. "Antioxidant and antiproliferative activities of common fruits." *J Agric Food Chem* 2002; 50: 7449–7454.

Suzuki R, Rylander-Rudqvist T, Ye W, et al. "Dietary fiber intake and risk of postmenopausal breast cancer defined by estrogen and progesterone receptor status: a prospective cohort study among Swedish women." *Int J Cancer* 2008 Jan 15; 122(2): 403–412.

The Fourth International Fructan Symposium, Arolla, Switzerland, 16–20 Aug 2000.

Toba M, Okamatsu H, Shimizu S, et al. "Inhibition by apple polyphenols of adp-ribosyltransferase activity of cholera toxin and toxin-induced fluid accumulation in mice." *Microbiology and Immunology* 2002; 46(4): 249–255,

Varma SD, Mizuno A, Kinoshita JH. "Diabetic cataracts and flavonoids." *Sci* 1977; 195: 205–206,

Vinson J, Su X, Zubik L, et al. "Phenol antioxidant quantity and quality in foods: fruits." *J Agric Food Chem* 2001; 49: 5315–5321.

Wolfe K, Wu X and Liu RH. "Antioxidant activity of apple peels." *J Agric Food Chem* 2003; 51: 609–614.

Baker BP, Benbrock CM, Groth E, et al. "Pesticide residues in conventional IPM-grown and organic foods: Insights from three U.S. data sets." *Food Additives and Contaminants* 2002 May; 19(5): 427–446.

Apricots

Aldoori WH, Giovannucci EL, Rockett H, et al. "A prospective study of dietary fiber types and symptomatic diverticular disease in men." *J Nutr* 1998 Apr 1; 128(4): 714–719.

Anderson JW. "Dietary fiber, lipids and atherosclerosis." *Am J Cardiol* 1987 Oct 30; 60(12): 17G–22G.

Cho E, Seddon JM, Rosner B, et al. "Prospective study of intake of fruits, vegetables, vitamins, and carotenoids and risk of age-related maculopathy." *Arch Ophthalmol* 2004 Jun; 122(6): 883–892.

Bingham SA, Day NE, Luben R, et al. "Dietary fibre in food and protection against colorectal cancer in the European Prospective Investigation into Cancer and Nutrition (EPIC): an observational study." *Lancet* 2003 May; 361(9368): 1496–1501.

Wald NJ, Thompson SG, Denson JW, et al. "Serum beta-carotene and subsequent risk of cancer: results from the BUPA study." *Br J Cancer* 1988; 57: 428–433.

Kritchevsky SB "Beta-carotene, carotenoids and the prevention of coronary heart disease." *J Nutr* 1999 Jan; 129(1): 5–8.

Suzuki K, Ito Y, Nakamura S, et al. "Relationship between serum carotenoids and hyperglycemia: a population-based cross-sectional study." *J Epidemiol* 2002 Sept; 12(5): 357–366.

Firth W and Norman R. "The effects of modified diets on urinary risk factors for kidney stone disease." *J Canadian Diet Assoc* 1990; 51(3): 404–408.

"Fruit Fights Infertility." All India Institute of Medical Sciences study reported in *BBC News Online,* December 18, 2000.

Hankinson SE, Stampfer MJ, Seddon JM, et al. "Nutrient intake and cataract extraction in women: a prospective study." *BMJ* 1992; 305(6849): 335–339.

Harris WS. "The prevention of atherosclerosis with antioxidants." *Clin Cardiol* 1992 Sep; 15(9): 636–640.

Hirvonen T, Virtanen M, Pietinen P. "Nutrient intake and use of beverages and the risk of kidney stones among male smokers." *Am J Epidemiol* 1999; 150(2): 187–194.

Shariati A, Maceda J, Hale D. "High-fiber diet for treatment of constipation in women with pelvic floor disorders." *Obstetrics and Gynecology* 2008; 111(4): 908–913.

References

Jian L, Lee AH, Binns CW. "Tea and lycopene protect against prostate cancer." *Asia Pac J Clin Nutri* 2007; 16 (Suppl 1): 453–457.

Klein R, et al. "Glycosylated hemoglobin in a population-based study of diabetes." *Am J Epidemiol* 1987; 126: 415–428.

Kuhad A, Seth R, Chopa K. "Lycopene attenuates diabetes associated cognitive decline in rats." *Life Sci* 2008 Jul 18; 83(3–4): 128–134.

Mayo Clinic. "Lycopene (high blood pressure, breast cancer, sun protection, prostate cancer, gingivitis)." Available online at: www.mayoclinic.com/health/lycopene/NS_patient-lycopene.

McCarty M, Waugh R, Ludwig D, et al. "Dietary fiber and weight gain." *JAMA* 2000; 283(14): 1821–1822.

Palan P and Naz R. "Changes in various antioxidant levels in human seminal plasma related to immunoinfertility." *Arch Androl* 1996 Mar–Apr; 36(2): 139–143

Seddon JM, et al. "Dietary carotenoids, vitamins A, C, and E, and advanced age-related macular degeneration." *JAMA* 1994 Nov 9; 272: 1413–1420.

Arugula

Cohen JH, et al. "Fruit and vegetable intakes and prostate cancer." *J Natl Cancer Insti* 2000; 92(1): 61–68.

Gilbert S, et al. "Effects of a combination of beta-carotene and vitamin A on lung cancer and cardiovascular disease." *N Engl J Med* 1996; 334(18): 1150–1155.

Jacques PF, Selhub J, Bostom AG, et al. "The effect of folic acid fortification on plasma folate and total homocysteine concentrations." *N Engl J Med* 1999; 340: 1449–1454.

Snodderly DM. "Evidence for protection against age-related macular degeneration by carotenoids and antioxidant vitamins." *Am J Clin Nutr* 1995; 62 (Suppl): 1448S–1461S.

National Eye Institute, National Instisutes of Health. "Lutein and its role in eye disease prevention." NEI Statement, 2002 Jul. Available online at: www.nei.nih.gov/news/statements/lutein/htm.

Teikari JM, Virtamo J, Rautalahti M, et al. "Long-term supplementation with alpha-tocopherol and beta-carotene and age-related cataract." *Acta Ophthalmol Scand* 1997; 75: 634–640.

Zhang SM, Hunter DJ, Rosner BA. "Intakes of fruits, vegetables, and related nutrients and the risk of Non-Hodgkin's lymphoma among women." *Cancer Epidemiology Biomarkers & Prevention* 2000 May; 9: 477–485.

Hara M, Hanaoka T, et al. "Cruciferous vegetables, mushrooms, and gastrointestinal cancer risks in a multicenter, hospital-based case-control study in Japan." *Nutrition and Cancer* 2003 Jul 2; 46(2): 138–147.

University of California-Berkeley. "Genetic abnormalities in sperm linked to dietary folate intake, study shows." *ScienceDaily.com* 2008 Mar 20. Available online at: www.sciencedaily.com/releases/2008/03/080319193036.htm.

Keck AS and Finley JW. "Cruciferous vegetables: cancer protective mechanisms of glucosinolate hydrolysis products and selenium." *Integrative Cancer Therapies* 2004; 3(1): 5–12.

Science Daily. "Properties in cruciferous veggies." *ScienceDaily.com*. Available online at: www.sciencedaily.com /releases/2007/05/070517100315.htm.

Asparagus

American Diabetes Association. *Diabetes* 1991; 40(3): 344–348.

Arikan S, Akcay T, Konukoglu D, et al. "The relationship between antioxidant enzymes and bladder cancer." *Neoplasma* 2005; 52(4): 314–317.

Boyle SP, Dobson VL, Duthie SJ, et al. "Bioavailability and efficiency of rutin as an antioxidant: A human supplementation study." *EJCN* 2000 Oct; 54(10): 774–782.

Cario-Toumaniantz C, Boularan C, Schurgers, LJ, et al. "Identification of differentially expressed genes in human varicose veins: Involvement of matrix gla protein in extracellular matrix remodeling." *J Vascular Res* 2007 Jul 20; 44(6): 444–459.

Cesarone MR, Incandela L, DeSanctis MT, et al. "Treatment of edema and increased capillary filtration in venous hypertension with HR (Paroven, Venoruton; 0-[beta-hydroxyethyl]-rutosides): a clinical, prospective, placebo-controlled, randomized, dose-ranging trial." *J Cardiovasc Pharmacol Ther* 2002 Jan; 7 (Suppl 1): S21–S24.

Cesarone MR, Incandela L, DeSanctis MT, et al. "Variations in plasma free radicals in patients with venous hypertension with HR (Paroven, Venoruton; 0-[beta-hydroxyethyl]-rutosides): A clinical, prospective, placebo-controlled, randomized trial." *J Cardiovasc Pharmacol Ther* 2002 Jan; 7 (Suppl 1): S25–S28.

Christen WG, Glynn RJ, Chow EY, et al. "Folic acid, pyridoxine, and cyanocobalamin combination treatment and age-related macular degeneration in women." *Arch Intern Med* 2009 Feb 23; 169(4): 335–341.

Cohen SM, Olin KL, Feuer WJ, et al. "Low glutathione reductase and peroxidase activity in age-related macular degeneration." *Br J Ophthalmol* 1994 Oct; 78(10): 791–794.

European Journal of Clinical Nutrition Advance online publication; doi: 10.1038/sj.ejcn.1602636

Huang HS, Ma MC, and Chen J. "Low vitamin E diet exacerbates calcium oxalate crystal formation via enhanced oxidative stress in rat hyperoxaluric kidney." *Am J Physiol Renal Physiol* 2009 Jan; 296(1): F34–F45.

Incandela L, Cesarone MR, DeSanctis MT, et al. "Treatment of diabetic microangiopathy and edema with HR (Paroven, Venoruton; 0-[beta-hydroxyethyl]-rutosides): A prospective, placebo-controlled, randomized study." *J Cardiovasc Pharmacol Ther* 2002 Jan; 7 (Suppl 1): S11–S15.

Kaynar H, Meral M, Turhan H, et al. "Glutathione peroxidase, glutathione-S-transferase, catalase, xanthine oxidase, Cu-Zn superoxide dismutase activities, total glutathione, nitric oxide, and malondialdehyde levels in erythrocytes of patients with small cell and non-small cell lung cancer." *Cancer Lett.* 2005 Sep 28; 227(2): 133–139.

Kim LS, Axelrod LJ, Howard P, et al. "Efficacy of methylsulfonylmethane (MSM) in osteoarthritis pain of the knee: a pilot clinical trial." *Osteoarthritis Cartilage* 2006 Mar; 14(3): 286–294.

Matthews GM and Butler RN. "Cellular mucosal defense during *Helicobacter pylori* infection: a review of the role of glutathione and the oxidative pentose pathway." *Helicobacter* 2005 Aug; 10(4): 298–306.

Mayo Clinic. "Arginine." *MayoClinic.com* (2010 Jun 1). Available online at: www.mayoclinic.com/health/l-arginine/NS_patient-arginine.

Murray-Kolb LE, et al. "Iron treatment normalizes cognitive functioning in young women." *Am J Clin Nutr,* 2007; 85(3): 778–787.

Onoda H, Takahashi H, Osada M, et al. "The relationship between the intracellular redox status of immune cells and progression of hepatitis C virus related chronic liver disease." [Article in Japanese] *Nihon Rinsho Meneki Gakkai Kaishi* 2004 Oct; 27(5): 315–321.

Petruzzellis V, Troccoli T, Candiani C, et al. "Oxerutins (venoruton): efficacy in chronic venous insufficiency—a double-blind, randomized, controlled study." *Angiology* 2002 May–Jun; 53(3): 257–263.

Rajbhandari M, Mentel R, Jha PK, et al. "Antiviral activity of some plants used in Nepalese traditional medicine." CCAM 2009; 6(4): 517–522.

Rieder M. "Prevention of neural tube defects with periconceptional folic acid." *Clin Perinatol* 1994; 21: 483–502.

Science News. "How effective are probiotics in irritable bowel syndrome?" *ScienceDaily.com* 2008, Oct 10. Available online at: www.sciencedaily.com/releases/2008/10/081006092656.htm.

Shearer MJ. "The roles of vitamins D and K in bone health and osteoporosis prevention." *Proc Nutr Soc* 1997; 56(3): 915–937.

Shimizu H, Kiyohara Y, Kato I, et al. "Relationship between plasma glutathione levels and cardiovascular disease in a defined population: the Hisayama study." *Stroke* 2004 Sep; 35(9): 2072–2077.

References

Sims NR, Nilsson M, Muyderman H. "Mitochondrial glutathione: A modulator of brain cell death." *J Bioenerg Biomembr* 2004 Aug; 36(4): 329–333.

Titapant V, Indrasukhsri B, Lekprasert V, et al. "Trihydroxyethylrutosides in the treatment of hemorrhoids of pregnancy: a double-blind placebo-controlled trial." *J Med Assoc Thai* 2001 Oct; 84(10): 1395–1400.

Visavadiya NP, et al. "Asparagus root regulates cholesterol metabolism and improves antioxidant status in hypercholesteremic rats." *ECAM* 2009; 6(2): 219-226

Yeh CC, Hou MF, Wu SH, et al. "A study of glutathione status in the blood and tissues of patients with breast cancer." *Cell Biochem Funct* 2005 Sep 2; 24(6): 555–559.

Avocados

Aprahamian M, Dentinger A, Stock-Damge C, et al. "Effects of supplemental pantothenic acid on wound healing: experimental study in rabbit." *Am J Clin Nutr* 1985; 41(3): 578–589.

Bazzano LA, He J, Odgen LG, et al. "Dietary intake of folate and risk of stroke in US men and women: NHANES I epidemiologic follow-up study." *Stroke* 2002 May; 33(5): 1183–1189.

Carpenter TO, DeLucia MC, Zhang JH, et al. "A randomized controlled study of effects of dietary magnesium oxide supplementation on bone mineral content in healthy girls." *JCEM* 2006; 91(12): 4866–4872.

Cosgrove, MC, Franco OH, Granger SP, et al. "Dietary nutrient intakes and skin-aging appearance among middle-aged American women." *Am J Clin Nutr* 2007 Oct; 86: 1225–1231.

Ding H, Chin YW, Kinghorn AD, et al. "Chemopreventive characteristics of avocado fruit." *Semin Cancer Biol* 2007 Oct; 17(5): 386–394.

Lopez-Ledesma R, Frati-Munari AC, Hernandez-Dominguez BC, et al. "Monounsaturated fatty acid (avocado) rich diet for mild hypercholesterolemia." *Arch Med Res* 1996 Winter; 27(4): 519–523.

Lu QY, Arteaga JR, Zhang Q, et al. "Inhibition of prostate cancer cell growth by an avocado extract: role of lipid-soluble bioactive substances." *J Nutr Biochem* 2005 Jan; 16(1): 23–30.

Rimm EB, et al. "Folate and vitamin B_6 from diet and supplementation in relation to risk of coronary heart disease among women." *JAMA* 1998; 279(5): 359–364.

Shearer MJ. "The roles of vitamins D and K in bone health and osteoporosis prevention." *Proc Nutr Soc* 1997; 56(3): 915–937.

Unlu NZ, Bohn T, Clinton SK, et al. "Carotenoid absorption from salad and salsa by humans is enhanced by the addition of avocado or avocado oil." *J Nutr* 2005 Mar; 135(3): 431–436.

Walker A, De Souza M, Vickers M, et al. "Magnesium supplementation alleviates premenstrual symptoms of fluid retention." *J Womens Health* 1998 Nov; 7(9): 1157–1165.

Bananas

Ascherio A, Rimm EB, Hernan MA, et al. "Intake of potassium, magnesium, calcium, and fiber and risk of stroke among US men." *Circulation* 1998 Sep 22; 98(12):1198–1204.

Bazzano LA, He J, Ogden LG, et al. "Dietary fiber intake and reduced risk of coronary heart disease in US men and women: the National Health and Nutrition Examination Survey I Epidemiologic Follow-up Study." *Arch Intern Med* 2003 Sep 8; 163(16): 1897–1904.

Cho E, Seddon JM, Rosner B, et al. "Prospective study of intake of fruits, vegetables, vitamins, and carotenoids and risk of age-related maculopathy." *Arch Ophthalmol* 2004 Jun; 122(6): 883–892.

Dunjic BS, Svensson I, Axelson J, et al. "Green banana protection of gastric mucosa against experimentally induced injuries in rats: a multicomponent mechanism." *Scand J Gastroenterol* 1993 Oct; 28(10): 894–898.

Englberger L, Darnton-Hill I, Coyne T, et al. "Carotenoid-rich bananas: a potential food source for alleviating vitamin A deficiency." *Food Nutr Bull* 2003 Dec; 24(4): 303–318.

Mousain-Bosc M, Roche M, Polge A, et al. "Improvement of neurobehavioral disorders in children supplemented with magnesium-vitamin B$_6$. I. Attention deficit hyperactivity disorders." *Magnesium Research* 2006 Mar; 19(1): 53–62.

Rabbani GH, Teka T, Saha SK, et al. "Green banana and pectin improve small intestinal permeability and reduce fluid loss in Bangladeshi children with persistent diarrhea." *Dig Dis Sci* 2004 Mar; 49(3): 475–484.

Rao NM. "Protease inhibitors from ripened and unripened bananas." *Biochem Int* 1991 May; 24(1): 13–22.

Rashidkhani B, Lindblad P, Wolk A. "Fruits, vegetables and risk of renal cell carcinoma: a prospective study of Swedish women." *Int J Cancer* 2005 Jan 20; 113(3): 451–455.

Sellmeyer DE, Schloetter DE, Schloetter M, et al. "Potassium citrate prevents urine calcium excretion and bone resorption induced by a high sodium chloride diet." *J Clin Endo Metab* 2002; 87(5): 2008–2012.

Beets

"Need a remedy to help fight your PMS?" *Health on Today* 2007 Jun 24. Available online at: today .msnbc.msn.com/id/19405047.

Bobek P, Galbavy S, Mariassyova M. "The effect of red beet (*Beta vulgaris* var. *rubra*) fiber on alimentary hypercholesterolemia and chemically induced colon carcinogenesis in rats." *Nahrung* 2000 Jun; 44(3): 184–187.

Detopoulou P, Panagiotakos DB, Antonopoulou S, et al. "Dietary choline and betaine intakes in relation to concentrations of inflammatory markers in healthy adults: the ATTICA study." *Am J Clin Nutr* 2008 Feb; 87(2): 424–430. 2008.

Genco R. "Vitamin C deficiency increases risk for gum disease." *Periodontology* 2000 Aug 16; 71(8): 1215–1223.

Ilnitskii AP and Iurchenko VA. "Effect of fruit and vegetable juices on the changes in the production of carcinogenic N-nitroso compounds in human gastric juice." *Vopr Pitan* 1993 Jul–Sep; (4): 44–46.

Nagai T, Ishizuka S, Hara H, et al. "Dietary sugar beet fiber prevents the increase in aberrant crypt foci induced by gamma-irradiation in the colorectum of rats treated with an immunosuppressant." *J Nutr* 2000 Jul; 130(7): 1682–1687.

Olthof MR, van Vliet T, Boelsma E, et al. "Low-dose betaine supplementation leads to immediate and long-term lowering of plasma homocysteine in healthy men and women." *J Nutr* 2003 Dec; 133(12): 4135–4138.

Black Beans

Azevedo L, Gomes JC, Stringheta PC, et al. "Black bean (*Phaseolus vulgaris L.*) as a protective agent against DNA damage in mice." *Food Chem Toxicol* 2003 Dec; 41(12): 1671–1676.

Bazzano LA, He J, Ogden LG, et al. "Dietary fiber intake and reduced risk of coronary heart disease in US men and women: the NHANES I Epidemiologic Follow-up Study." *Arch Intern Med* 2003 Sep 8; 163(16): 1897–1904.

Karlsen A, Retterstol L, Laake P, et al. "Authocyanins inhibit nuclear factor kb activation in monocytes and reduce plasma concentrations of pro-inflammatory mediators in healthy adults." *J Nutr* 2007 Aug; 137: 1951–1954.

Ensminger AH, Ensminger ME, Kondale JE, et al. *Foods & Nutrition Encyclopedia.* Clovis, CA: Pegus Press, 1983.

Jing P, Bomser JA, Schwartz SJ, et al. "Structure-function relationships of anthocyanins from various anthocyanin-rich extracts on the inhibition of colon cancer cell growth." *J Agric Food Chem* 2008 Oct 22; 56(20): 9391–9398.

Lagiou P, Rossi M, Lagiou A, et al. "Flavonoid intake and liver cancer: a case-control study in Greece." *Cancer Causes Control* 2008 Oct; 19(8): 813–818.

Tsuda T. "Regulation of adipocyte function by anthocyanins; possibility of preventing the metabolic syndrome." *J Agric Food Chem* 2008; 56(3): 642–646.

Blueberries

Andres-Lacueva C, Shukitt-Hale B, Galli RL, et al. "Anthocyanins in aged blueberry-fed rats are found centrally and may enhance memory." *Nutr Neurosci* 2005 Apr; 8(2): 111–120.

USDA/ARS. "Mechanisms involved in the beneficial effects of blueberries on neuronal aging and behavior. Findings in *Nutritional Neuroscience*. Available online at: www.ars.usda.gov/research/projects/projects.htm?ACCN_NO=410302.

Gates MA, Tworoger SS, Hecht JL, et al. "A prospective study of dietary flavonoid intake and incidence of epithelial ovarian cancer." *Int J Cancer* 2007 Nov 15; 121(10): 2225–2232.

Joseph JA, Shukitt-Hale B, Denisova NA, et al. "Reversals of age-related declines in neuronal signal transduction, cognitive, and motor behavioral deficits with blueberry, spinach, or strawberry dietary supplementation." *J Neurosci* 1999 Sept 15; 19(18): 8114–8121.

Shukitt-Hale B, Carey AN, Jenkins D, et al. "Beneficial effects of fruit extracts on neuronal function and behavior in a rodent model of accelerated aging." *Neurobiol Aging* 2006 Jul 10; 28(8): 1187–1194.

Broccoli

Beecher C. "Cancer preventive properties of varieties of Brassica oleracea: a review." *Am J Clin Nutr* 1994; 59 (Suppl): 1166S–1170S.

Canene-Adams K, Lindshield BL, Wang S, et al. "Combinations of tomato and broccoli enhance antitumor activity in dunning r3327-h prostate adenocarcinomas." *Cancer Res* 2007 Jan 15; 67(2): 836–843.

Cohen JH, Kristal AR, et al. "Fruit and vegetable intakes and prostate cancer risk." *J Natl Cancer Inst* 2000 Jan 5; 92(1): 61–68.

Dinkova-Kostova AT, Jenkins SN, Fahey JW, et al. "Protection against UV-light-induced skin carcinogenesis in SKH-1 high-risk mice by sulforaphane-containing broccoli sprout extracts." *Cancer Lett* 2005 Nov 2; 240: 243–52.

Fahey JW, Haristoy X, Dolan PM, et al. "Sulforaphane inhibits extracellular, intracellular, and antibiotic-resistant strains of *Helicobacter pylori* and prevents benzopyrene-induced stomach tumors." *Proc Natl Acad Sci USA* 2002 May 28; 99(11): 7610–7615.

Fahey JW, Zhang Y, Talalay P. "Broccoli sprouts: an exceptionally rich source of inducers of enzymes that protect against chemical carcinogens." *Proc Natl Acad Sci USA* 1997 Sept 16; 94(19): 10367–10372.

Gates MA, Tworoger SS, Hecht JL, et al. "A prospective study of dietary flavonoid intake and incidence of epithelial ovarian cancer." *Int J Cancer* 2007 Apr 30; 121(10): 2225–2232.

Haristoy X, Angioi-Duprez K, Duprez A, et al. "Efficacy of sulforaphane in eradicating *Helicobacter pylori* in human gastric xenografts implanted in nude mice." *Antimicrob Agents Chemother* 2003 Dec; 47(12): 3982–3984.

Huxley RR and Neil HAW. "The relation between dietary flavonol intake and coronary heart disease mortality: a meta-analysis of prospective cohort studies." *Eur J Clin Nutr* 2003; 57: 904–908.

Jackson SJ and Singletary KW. "Sulforaphane inhibits human mcf-7 mammary cancer cell mitotic progression and tubulin polymerization." *J Nutr* 2004 Sep; 134(9): 2229–2236.

Kirsh VA, Peters U, Mayne ST, et al. "Prostate, lung, colorectal and ovarian cancer screening trial: prospective study of fruit and vegetable intake and risk of prostate cancer." *J Natl Cancer Inst* 2007 Aug 1; 99(15): 1200–1209.

Meng Q, Goldberg ID, Rosen EM, et al. "Inhibitory effects of indole-3-carbinol on invasion and migration in human breast cancer cells." *Breast Cancer Res Treat* 2000 Sep; 63(2): 147–152.

Nestle M. "Broccoli sprouts as inducers of carcinogen-detoxifying enzyme systems: clinical, dietary, and policy implications." *Proc Natl Acad Sci USA* 1997 Oct 14; 94(21): 11149–11151.

Pattison DJ, Silman AJ, Goodson NJ, et al. "Vitamin C and the risk of developing inflammatory polyarthritis: prospective nested case-control study." *Ann Rheum Dis* 2004 Jul; 63(7): 843–847.

Thys-Jacobs S, Starkey P, Bernstein D, et al. "Calcium carbonate and the premenstrual syndrome: effects on premenstrual and menstrual symptoms." Premenstrual syndrome study group. *Am J Obstet Gynecol* 1998; 179(2): 444–452.

Voorrips LE, Goldbohm RA, et al. "Vegetable and fruit consumption and risks of colon and rectal cancer in a prospective cohort study: The Netherlands Cohort Study on Diet and Cancer." *Am J Epidemiol* 2000 Dec 1; 152(11): 1081–1092.

Wu L, Ashraf MH, Facci M, et al. "Dietary approach to attenuate oxidative stress, hypertension, and inflammation in the cardiovascular system." *Proc Natl Acad Sci USA* 2004 May 4; 101(18): 7094–7099.

Yanaka A, Zhang S, Tauchi M, et al. "Role of the nrf-2 gene in protection and repair of gastric mucosa against oxidative stress." *Inflammopharmacology* 2005; 13(1–3): 83–90.

Yurtsever E and Yardimci KT. "The in vivo effect of a *Brassica oleracea* var. *capitata* extract on Ehrlich ascites tumors of MUS musculus BALB/C mice." *Drug Metabol Drug Interact* 1999; 15(2–3): 215–222.

Zhang J, Hsu BAJ, Kinseth BA, et al. "Indole-3-carbinol induces a G1 cell cycle arrest and inhibits prostate-specific antigen production in human LNCaP prostate carcinoma cells." *Cancer* 2003 Dec 1; 98(11): 2511–2520.

Zhang Y, Kensler TW, Cho CG, et al. "Anticarcinogenic activities of sulforaphane and structurally related synthetic norbornyl isothiocyanates." *Proc Natl Acad Sci USA* 1994 Apr 12; 91(8): 3147–3150.

Zhao B, Seow A, et al. "Dietary isothiocyanates, glutathione S-transferase -M1, -T1 polymorphisms and lung cancer risk among Chinese women in Singapore." *Cancer Epidemiol Biomarkers Prev* 2001 Oct; 10(10): 1063–1067.

Zhao H, Lin J, Grossman HB, et al. "Dietary isothiocyanates, GSTM1, GSTT1, NAT2 polymorphisms and bladder cancer risk." *Int J Cancer* 2007 May 15; 120(10): 2208–2213.

Cabbage

Beecher C. "Cancer preventive properties of varieties of *Brassica oleracea:* a review." *Am J Clin Nutr* 1994; 59 (Suppl): 1166S–1170S.

Brooks JD, Paton VG, Vidanes G. "Potent induction of phase 2 enzymes in human prostate cells by sulforaphane." *Cancer Epidemiol Biomarkers Prev* 2001 Sep; 10(9): 949–954.

Cheney G. "Anti-peptic ulcer dietary factor." *J Am Diet Assoc* 1950; 26: 668–672.

Cheney G. "Rapid healing of peptic ulcers in patients receiving fresh cabbage juice." *Cal Med* 1949; 70: 10–14.

Cohen JH, Kristal AR, et al. "Fruit and vegetable intakes and prostate cancer risk." *J Natl Cancer Inst* 2000 Jan 5; 92(1): 61–68.

Fowke JH, Chung FL, Jin F, et al. "Urinary isothiocyanate levels, brassica, and human breast cancer." *Cancer Res* 2003 Jul 15; 63(14): 3980–3986.

Heo HJ and Chang YL. "Phenolic phytochemicals in cabbage inhibit amyloid beta protein-induced neurotoxicity." *Food Science and Technology* 2006 May; 39(4): 331–337.

Hu R, Khor TO, Shen G, et al. "Cancer chemoprevention of intestinal polyposis in ApcMin/+ mice by sulforaphane, a natural product derived from cruciferous vegetable." *Carcinogenesis* 2006 Oct; 27(10): 2038–2046.

Jackson SJ and Singletary KW. "Sulforaphane inhibits human mcf-7 mammary cancer cell mitotic progression and tubulin polymerization." *J Nutr* 2004 Sept; 134(9): 2229–2236.

Johnson IT. "Glucosinolates: bioavailability and importance to health." *Int J Vitam Nutr Res* 2002 Jan; 72(1): 26–31.

References

Johnson IT. "Vegetables yield anticancer chemical." Institute of Food Research, News Release, 10 May 2004. Available online at: www.ifr.ac.uk.

Kawamori T, Tanaka T, Ohnishi M, et al. "Chemoprevention of azoxymethane-induced colon carcinogenesis by dietary feeding of S-methyl methane thiosulfonate in male F344 rats." *Cancer Res* 1995 Sep 15; 55(18): 4053–4058.

Kurilich AC, Tsau GJ, Brown A, et al. "Carotene, tocopherol, and ascorbate contents in subspecies of *Brassica oleracea*." *J Agric Food Chem* 1999 Apr; 47(4): 1576–1581.

Kwak MK, Egner PA, Dolan PM, et al. "Role of phase 2 enzyme induction in chemoprotection by dithiolethiones." *Mutat Res* 2001 Sep 1; 480–481: 305–315.

Maiyoh GK, Kuh JE, Casaschi A, et al. "Cruciferous indole-3-carbinol inhibits apolipoprotein B secretion in HepG2 cells." *J Nutr* 2007 Oct; 137(10): 2185–2189.

Michnovicz JJ and Bradlow HL. "Altered estrogen metabolism and excretion in humans following consumption of indole-3-carbinol." *Nutr Cancer* 1991; 16(1): 59–66.

Pathak DR, et al. "Joint association of high cabbage/sauerkraut intake at 12–13 years of age and adulthood with reduced breast cancer risk in Polish migrant women: results from the US component of the Polish women's health study (PWHS)." Abstract #3697. Presented at the AACR 4th Annual Conference on Frontiers in Cancer Prevention Research, October 30–November 2, 2005, Baltimore, MD.

Shive W, Snider RN, DuBiler B, et al. "Glutamine in treatment of peptic ulcer." *Tex J Med* 1957; 53: 840–843.

Siddiqi M, Tricker AR, Preussmann R. "Formation of N-nitroso compounds under simulated gastric conditions from Kashmir foodstuffs." *Cancer Lett* 1988 Apr; 39(3): 259–265.

Steinkellner H, Rabot S, Freywald C, et al. "Effects of cruciferous vegetables and their constituents on drug metabolizing enzymes involved in the bioactivation of DNA-reactive dietary carcinogens." *Mutat Res* 2001 Sep 1; 480–481: 285–297.

Stoewsand GS. "Bioactive organosulfur phytochemicals in *Brassica oleracea* vegetables—a review." *Food Chem Toxicol* 1995 Jun; 33(6): 537–43.

Thimmulappa RK, Mai KH, Srisuma S, et al. "Identification of Nrf2-regulated genes induced by the chemopreventive agent sulforaphane by oligonucleotide microarray." *Cancer Res* 2002 Sep 15; 62(18): 5196–5203.

Verhoeven DT, Goldbom RA, van Poppel G, et al. "Epidemiologcal studies on brassica vegetables and cancer risk." *Cancer Epidemiol Biomarkers Prev* 1996 Sep; 5(9): 773–748.

Vitamin C Foundation. "Vitamin C and collagen." In *Nutrition Against Disease* by Roger J. Williams. New York, NY: Bantam Books, 1971; 85–86 and *How to Live Longer and Feel Better* by Linus Pauling. New York, NY: Avon, 1987; 89–91. See also www.vitamincfoundation.org/collagen.html.

Yurtsever E and Yardimci KT. "The in vivo effect of a *Brassica oleracea* var. capitata extract on Ehrlich ascites tumors of MUS musculus BALB/C mice." *Drug Metabol Drug Interact* 1999; 15(2–3): 215–222.

Zhao B, Seow A, et al. "Dietary isothiocyanates, glutathione S-transferase -M1, -T1 polymorphisms and lung cancer risk among Chinese women in Singapore." *Cancer Epidemiol Biomarkers Prev* 2001 Oct; 10(10): 1063–1067.

Zhao H, Lin J, Grossman HB, et al. "Dietary isothiocyanates, GSTM1, GSTT1, NAT2 polymorphisms and bladder cancer risk." *Int J Cancer* 2007 May 15; 120(10): 2208–2213.

Carrots

Ensminger A. *Food for Health: A Nutrition Encyclopedia.* Clovis, CA: Pegus Press, 1986.

Gaziano JM, Manson JE, Branch LG, et al. "A prospective study of consumption of carotenoids in fruits and vegetables and decreased cardiovascular mortality in the elderly." *Ann Epidemiol* 1995; 5: 255–260.

Harris RA, Key TJ, Silcocks PB, et al. "A case-controlled study of dietary carotene in men with lung cancer and in men with other epithelial cancers." *Nutrition and Cancer* 199; 15: 63–68.

Kobaek-Larsen M, Christensen LP, Vach W, et al. "Inhibitory effects of feeding with carrots or (-)-falcarinol on development of azoxymethane-induced preneoplastic lesions in the rat colon." *J Agric Food Chem* 2005 Mar 9; 53(5): 1823–1827 [PMID: 15740080].

Li T, Molteni A, Latkovich P, et al. "Vitamin A depletion induced by cigarette smoke is associated with the development of emphysema in rats." *J Nutr* 2003 Aug; 133(8): 2629–2634 [PMID: 12888649].

Michaud DS, Feskanich D, Rimm EB, et al. "Intake of specific carotenoids and risk of lung cancer in 2 prospective US cohorts." *Am J Clin Nutr* 2000 Oct; 72(4): 990–997.

Natural Environment Research Council. "Could carrots be the secret to a long life and sex appeal?" *ScienceDaily.* www.sciencedaily.com /releases/2007/05/070510105549.htm (retrieved Aug 18, 2008).

Nicolle C, Cardinault N, Aprikian O, et al. "Effect of carrot intake on cholesterol metabolism and on antioxidant status in cholesterol-fed rat." *Eur J Nutr* 2003 Oct; 42(5): 254–261.

Wald NJ, Thompson SG, Densem JW, et al. "Serum beta-carotene and subsequent risk of cancer: results from the BUPA study." *Br J Cancer* 1988; 57: 428–433.

Wood R. *The Whole Foods Encyclopedia.* NY, NY: Prentice-Hall Press, 1988 [PMID: 15220].

Ylonen K, Alfthan G, Groop L, et al. "Dietary intakes and plasma concentrations of carotenoids and tocopherols in relation to glucose metabolism in subjects at high risk of type 2 diabetes: the Botnia Dietary Study." *Am J Clin Nutr* 2003 Jun; 77(6): 1434–1441.

Cherries

Connolly DA, McHugh MP, Padilla-Zakour OI. "Efficacy of tart cherry juice blend in preventing the symptoms of muscle damage." *Br J Sports Med* online, June 21, 2006; 40: 679–683.

Davis JM, Murphy EA, McClellan JL, et al. "Quercetin reduces susceptibility to influenza infection following stressful exercise." *Am J Physiol Regul Integr Comp Physiol* 2008; 295: R505–R509.

Erlund I. "Review of the flavonoids quercetin, hesperetin, and naringenin: dietary sources, bioactives, bioavailability and epidemiology." *Nutr Res* 2004; 24: 851–874.

Falsaperla M, Morgia G, Tartarone A, et al. "Support ellagic acid therapy in patients with hormone refractory prostate cancer (HRPC) on standard chemotherapy using vinorelbine and estramustine phosphate." *Eur Urol* 2004 Apr; 47(4): 449–454; discussion 454–455.

Herxheimer A and Petrie KJ. "Melatonin for preventing and treating jet lag." *Cochrane Database Syst Rev* 2002; (2): CD001520. Review.

Jacob RA, Spinozzi GM, Simon VA "Consumption of cherries lowers plasma urate in healthy women." *Journal of Nutrition* 2003 Jun; 133: 1826–1829.

Kelley DS, Rasooly R, Jacob RA, et al. "Consumption of bing sweet cherries lowers circulating concentrations of inflammation markers in healthy men and women." *J Nutr* 2006; 136: 981–986.

Kim DO, Heo HJ, Kim YJ, et al. "Sweet and sour cherry phenolics and their protective effects on neuronal cells." *J Agric Food Chem* 2005; 53: 9921–9927.

Lewy AJ, Bauer VK, Cutler NL, et al. "Melatonin treatment of winter depression: a pilot study." *Psychiatry Res* 1998 Jan 16; 77(1): 57–61.

Matalas AL, Zampelas A, Stavrinos (eds). *The Mediterranean Diet: Constituents and Health Promotion.* Boca Raton, FL: CRC Press Modern Nutrition Series, 2001.

Reiter RJ, Tan DX, Osuna C, et al. "Actions of melatonin in the reduction of oxidative stress." *J Biomed Sci* 2000; 7: 444–458.

Tall JM, Seeram NP, Zhao C, et al. "Tart cherry anthocyanins suppress inflammation-induced pain behavior in rat." *Behav Brain Res* 2004; 153(1): 181–8.

References

Wade AG, Ford I, Crawford G, et al. "Efficacy of prolonged release melatonin in insomnia patients aged 55-80 years: quality of sleep and next-day alertness outcomes." *Curr Med Res Opin* 2007 Oct; 23(10): 2597–2605.

Chili Peppers

Ahuja KD and Ball MJ. "Effects of daily ingestion of chilli on serum lipoprotein oxidation in adult men and women." *Br J Nutr* 2006 Aug; 96(2): 239–242.

Ahuja KD, Robertson IK, Geraghty DP, et al. "Effects of chili consumption on postprandial glucose, insulin, and energy metabolism." *Am J Clin Nutr* 2006 Jul; 84(1): 63–69.

Attal N. "Chronic neuropathic pain: mechanisms and treatment." *Clin J Pain* 2000 Sep; 16 (Suppl 3): S118–S130.

Food Details. "Calories in Anaheim Chile." Calories Count. Available online at: http://caloriecount.about.com/calories-melissas-anaheim-chile-i115531.

Fusco BM, Marabini S, Maggi CA, et al. "Preventative effect of repeated nasal applications of capsaicin in cluster headache." *Pain* 1994 Dec; 59(3): 321–325.

Joe B and Lokesh BR. "Prophylactic and therapeutic effects of n-3 polyunsaturated fatty acids, capsaicin and curcumin on adjuvant induced arthritis in rats." *Nutr Biochem* 1997; 8: 397–407.

Johnston C, et al. "Antihistamine effect of supplemental ascorbic acid and neutrophil chemotaxis." *J Am Coll Nutr* 1992; 11: 172–176.

Kang JY, et al., "Chili-protective factor against peptic ulcer?" *Dig Dis Sci* 1995 Mar; 40: 576–579.

Marabinil S, Ciabatti PG, Polli G. "Beneficial effects of intranasal applications of capsaicin in patients with vasomotor rhinitis." *European Archives of Oto-Rhino-Laryngology* 1991 May; 248(4): 191–194.

Mauela P, Lejeune EH, Kovacs R. "Effect of capsaicin on substrate oxidation and weight maintenance after modest body-weight loss in human subjects." *Br J Nutr* 2003 Sep; 90(3): 651–659.

Mori A, Lehmann S, O'Kelly J, et al. "Capsaicin, a component of red peppers, inhibits the growth of androgen-independent, p53 mutant prostate cancer cells." *Cancer Res* 2006 Mar 15; 66(6): 3222–3229.

Schnitzer TJ. "Non-NSAID pharmacologic treatment options for the management of chronic pain." *Am J Med* 1998 Jul 27; 105(1B): 45S–52S.

Singh V, Schachter N, Hexter M. 100th International Conference of the American Thoracic Society, Orlando, FL, May 21–26, 2004.

Zhang J, Makoto N, Yuetsu T. "Capsaicin inhibits growth of adult T-cell leukemia cells." *Leuk Res* 2003 Mar; 27(3): 275–283.

Coffee

Brice CF and Smith AP. "Effects of caffeine on mood and performance: a study of realistic consumption." *Psychopharmacology* 2002; 164: 188–192.

Daglia M, Tarsi R, Papetti A. "Antiadhesive effect of green and roasted coffee on streptococcus mutans' adhesive properties on saliva-coated hydroxyapatite beads." *J Agric Food Chem* 2002 Feb 27; 50(5): 1225–1229.

Diamond S, Balm BS, Freitag FG. "Ibuprofen plus caffeine in the treatment of tension-type headaches." *Clin Pharmacol Ther* 2000; 68: 312–319.

Falk B, Burstein R, Rosenbloom J, et al. "Effects of caffeine ingestion on body fluid balance and thermoregulation during exercise." *Can J Physiol Pharmacol* 1990; 68(7): 889–892.

Fox M. "Coffee users at lower risk for Parkinson's study." *Reuters Life* 2007 Apr 9. Available online at: www.alertnet.org/thenews/newsdesk/N49334914.htm.

Gordon NF, Myburgh JL, Kruger PE, et al. "Effects of caffeine ingestion on thermoregulatory and myocardial function during endurance performance." *S Afr Med J* 1982; 62(18): 644–647.

Graham TE and Spiet LL. "Metabolic, catecholamine, and exercise performance responses to varying doses of caffeine." *J Appl Psyiol* 1995; 78: 867–874.

Kawachi I, et al. "A prospective study of coffee drinking and suicide in women." *Arch Intern Med* 1996; 156(5): 521–525.

Lindsay J, et al. "Risk factors for Alzheimer's disease: a prospective analysis from the Canadian study of health and aging." *Am J Epidemiol* 2002; 5: 445–453.

Lopez-Garcia E, van Dam R, Li TY, et al. "The relationship of coffee consumption with mortality." *Ann Intern Med* 2008 Jun 16; 148; 904–914.

Maia L, de Mendonca A. "Does caffeine intake protect from Alzheimer's disease?" *Eur J Neurol* 2002; 9(4): 377–382.

Pagano R, et al. "Coffee drinking and prevalence of bronchial asthma." *Chest* 1988; 94: 386–389.

Ramlau-Hansen CH, Thulstrup AM, Bonde JP. "Semen quality and present caffeine exposure: two decades of follow-up of a pregnancy cohort." *Hum Reprod* 2008; 23(12): 2799–2805.

Ruhl CE and Everhart JE. "Coffee and tea consumption are associated with a lower incidence of chronic liver disease in the United States." *Gastroenterology* 2005 Dec; 129(6): 1928–1936.

Smith B, et al. "Does coffee consumption reduce the risk of type 2 diabetes in individuals with impaired glucose?" *Diabetes Care* 2006 Nov; 29: 2385–2390.

Solinas M, Ferre S, You ZB, et al. "Caffeine induces dopamine and glutamate release in the shell of the nucleus accumbens." *J Neurosci* 2002 Aug 1; 22(15): 6321–6324

Van Dam R and Hu F. "Coffee consumption and risk of type 2 diabetes." *JAMA* 2005; 294: 97–104.

Warner J. "Drinking Lots of Coffee May Prevent Diabetes." *WebMD.com* 2004 Mar 9. Available online at: diabetes.webmd.com/news/20040309/drinking-coffee-prevent-diabetes.

Cucumbers

Appel LJ, Moore TJ, Obarzanek E, et al. "A clinical trial of the effects of dietary patterns on blood pressure." DASH Collaborative Research Group. *N Engl J Med* 1997 Apr 17; 336(16): 1117–1124.

Barel A, Calomme M, Timchenko A, et al. "Effect of oral intake of choline-stabilized orthosilicic acid on skin, nails and hair in women with photodamaged skin." *Arch Dermatol Res* 2005 Oct 5; 297(4): 147–153.

Bendich A. "The potential for dietary supplements to reduce premenstrual syndrome (PMS) symptoms." *J Am Coll Nut* 2000; 19(1): 3–11.

Carlisle EM. "Silicon as a trace nutrient." *Sci Total Environ* 1989; 73: 95–106.

Fillon M. "Silicon may play important role in bone health: presented at ASBMR." *Doctor's Guide* 2005 Sep 27; based on paper presented at the ASBMR 27th Annual Meeting (Sep 24, 2005). Paper title: "Effect on bone turnover and bmd of low dose oral silicon as an adjunct to calcium/vitamin d3 in a randomized, placebo-controlled trial." (Abstract SA421). Available online at: www.docguide.com/news/content.nsf/news/8525697700573 E188525708900574C94.

Rico H, Gallego-Lago JL, Hernandez ER, et al. "Effect of silicon supplement on osteopenia induced by ovariectomy in rats." *Calcif Tissue Int* 2000; 66: 53–55.

Seaborn CD and Nielsen FH. "Dietary silicon and arginine affect mineral element composition of rat femur and vertebra." *Biol Trace Elem Res* 2002 Dec; 89(3): 239–250.

Seaborn CD and Nielsen FH. "Silicon deprivation decreases collagen formation in wounds and bone, and ornithine transaminase enzyme activity in liver." *Biol Trace Elem Res.* 2002; 89: 251–261.

References

Wright J and Littleton K. "Defects in sulfur metabolism." *Internatl Clin Nut Rev* 1989; 9: 118–119.

Dark Chocolate

Aznaouridis K, et al. "Dark chocolate improves endothelial function and arterial stiffness in healthy individuals." American Heart Association Scientific Sessions, Chicago, 2004. Session Number/Title: AOP.41.1 *Nutrition and Cardiovascular Diseases,* Presentation Number 3584.

"Could a Chocolate a Day Stop Tooth Decay?" *Reuters* 2000 Aug 24.

Engler MB, Engler MM, and Chen CY. "Flavonoid-rich dark chocolate improves endothelial function and increases plasma epicatechin concentrations in healthy adults." *J Am Coll Nut* 2004; 23(3): 197–204.

Kondo K, Hirano R, Matsumoto A, et al. "Inhibition of LDL oxidation by cocoa." *Lancet* 1996 Nov; 348(2): 1514.

Lee IM and Paffenbarger R. "Life is sweet: candy consumption and longevity." *BMJ* 1998; 317: 1683–1684.

"Nutritional Functions of Cocoa and Chocolate." *The Manufacturing Confectioner* 2000 Feb: 2.

Polagruto JA, Wang-Polagruto JF, Braun MM., et al. "Cocoa flavanol-enriched snack bars containing phytosterols effectively lower total and LDL cholesterol levels." *J Am Diet Assoc* 2006 Nov; 106(11): 1804–1813.

Praag H. "Plant-derived flavonol epicatechin enhances angiogenesis and retention of spatial memory in mice." *J Neurosci* 2007 May 30; 27(22): 5869–5878.

Ramljak D, Romanczyk LJ. "Pentameric procyanidin from Theobroma cacao selectively inhibits growth of human breast cancer cells." *Journal Molecular Cancer Therapeutics,* 2005 Apr; 4(4): 537–546.

Tauber D. "Chocolate and blood pressure in elderly individuals with isolated systolic hypertension." *JAMA* 2003 Aug 27; 290 (8): 1029–1030.

Thijssen MA, Hornstra G, Mensink RP. "Stearic, oleic, and linoleic acids have comparable effects on markers of thrombotic tendency in healthy human subjects." *J Nutr* 2005; 135: 1805–1811.

Thys-Jacobs "Calcium carbonate and the premenstrual syndrome: effects on premensual and menstrual symptoms." *Am J Obst Gynecol* 1998 Aug; 179(2): 444–452.

Usmani OS, Beluisi MG, Patel HJ. "Theobromine inhibits sensory nerve activation and cough." *FASEB Journal* 2005 Feb; 19: 233.

Vinson JA, Proch J, Zubik L. "Phenol antioxidant quantity and quality in foods: cocoa, dark chocolate, and milk chocolate." *J Agric Food Chem* 1999 Dec; 47(12): 4821–4824.

Walker AF, DeSouza MC, Vickers MF. "Magnesium supplementation alleviates premenstrual symptoms of fluid retention." *J Womens Health* 1998; 7: 1157.

Zurer P. "Chocolate may mimic marijuana in brain." *Chem Eng News* 1996 Sep 2; 74: 31.

Dates

"Dietary potassium deficiency is independently associated with increased blood pressure in a multi-ethnic population-based cohort" (SA-FC404). Presented at the American Society of Nephrology's 41st Annual Meeting and Scientific Exposition, Nov 8, 2008, Philadelphia, PA.

Copper Development Association. Information for Consumers. Available online at: www.copper .org.

Demirkaya S, Vural O, Dora B, et al. "Efficacy of intravenous magnesium sulfate in the treatment of acute migraine attacks." *Headache* 2001; 41(2): 171–177.

Marano AE. "Vitamins: Busy Bs." *Psychology Today* 2004 Jul 26. Available online at: www.psychologytoday.com/articles/pto-20040726-000014.html.

Quaranta S, et al. "Pilot study of the efficacy and safety of a modified-release magnesium 250 mg tablet (Sincromag) for the treatment of premenstrual syndrome." *Clin Drug Investig* 2007; 27(1): 51–58.

Science News. "High potassium diet may protect against stroke." *ScienceDaily.com* 1998 Sep 23; Available online at: www.science daily.com/releases/1998/09/980923073215.htm.

Fennel

Chainy GB, Manna SK, Chaturvedi MM, et al. "Anethole blocks both early and late cellular responses transduced by tumor necrosis factor: effect on NF-kappaB, AP-1, JNK, MAPKK and apoptosis." *Oncogene* 2000 Jun 8; 19(25): 2943–2950.

Ensminger AH. *Food for Health: A Nutrition Encyclopedia.* Clovis, CA: Pegus Press, 1986.

Ensminger AH, Ensminger ME, Kondale JE, et al. *Foods & Nutrition Encyclopedia* (Vols 1 and 2). Clovis, CA: Pegus Press, 1983.

Ozbek H, Ugras S, Dulger H, et al. "Hepatoprotective effect of *Foeniculum vulgare* essential oil." *Fitoterapia* 2003 Apr; 74(3): 317–319.

Ruberto G, Baratta MT, Deans SG, et al. "Antioxidant and antimicrobial activity of *Foeniculum vulgare* and *Crithmum maritimum* essential oils." *Planta Med* 2000 Dec; 66(8): 687–693.

Figs

Cho E, Seddon JM, Rosner B, et al. "Prospective study of intake of fruits, vegetables, vitamins, and carotenoids and risk of age-related maculopathy." *Arch Ophthalmol* 2004 Jun; 122(6): 883–892.

Dobbyns S. *The Fertility Diet.* New York, NY: Simon & Schuster, 2008.

Harvard University. "Tamed 11,400 years ago, figs were likely first domesticated crop." *ScienceDaily.com* 2006 Jun 4. Available online at: www.sciencedaily.com/releases/2006/06/060602074522.htm.

Sellmeyer DE, Schloetter DE, Schloetter M, et al. "Potassium citrate prevents urine calcium excretion and bone resorption induced by a high sodium chloride diet." *J Clin Endo Metab* 2002; 87(5): 2008–2012.

Serraclara A, Hawkins F, Perez C, et al. "Hypoglycemic action of an oral fig-leaf decoction in type-I diabetic patients." *Diabetes Res Clin Pract* 1998 Jan; 39(1): 19–22.

Suzuki R, Rylander-Rudqvist T, Ye W, et al. "Dietary fiber intake and risk of postmenopausal breast cancer defined by estrogen and progesterone receptor status—a prospective cohort study among Swedish women." *Int J Cancer* 2008 Jan 15; 122(2): 403–412.

Vinson JA. *Cereal Foods World* 1999 Feb; a publication of the American Association of Cereal Chemists.

Wayatt K, Dimmock PW, Jones P. "Efficacy of vitamin B-6 in the treatment of premenstrual syndrome: systemic review." *BMJ* 1999 May 22; 318: 1375–1381.

Goji Berries

Amagase H and Nance D. "A randomized, double-blind, placebo-controlled, clinical study of the general effects of a standardized *Lycium barbarum* (Goji) juice, GoChi™." *JACM* 2008 May; 14(4): 403–412.

Cao GW, Yang WG, Du P. "Observation of the effects of LAK/IL-2 therapy combining with Lycium barbarum polysaccharides in the treatment of 75 cancer patients." *Zhonghua Zhong Liu Za Zhi* 1994 Nov; 16(6): 428–431 [Article in Chinese].

Deng HB, et al. "Inhibiting affects of Achyranthes bidentata polysaccharide and *Lycium barbarum* polysaccharide on nonenzyme glycation in D-galatose induced mouse aging model." *Biomed Environ Sci* 2003 Sep; 16(3): 267–275.

Gan L, Wang J and Zhang S. "Inhibition of the growth of human leukemia cells by *Lycium barbarum* polysaccharide." *Wei Sheng Yan Jiu* 2001 Nov; 30(6): 333–335 [Article in Chinese].

Huang X, Yang M, Wu X, et al. "Study on protective action of *Lycium barbarum* polysaccharides on DNA impairments of testicle cells in mice." *Wei Sheng Yan Jiu* 2003 Nov; 32(6): 599–601.

Kim SY, et al. "New antihepatotoxic cerebroside from Lycium chinense fruits." *J Nat Prod* 1997 Mar; 60(3); 274–276.

Snellen EL, Verbeek AL, Van Den Hoogen GW, et al. "Neovascular age-related macular degeneration and its relationship to antioxidant intake." *Acta Ophthalmol Scand* 2002 Aug; 80(4): 368–371.

Wu H, Guo H, Zhao R. "Effect of *Lycium barbarum* polysaccharide on the improvement of antioxidant ability and DNA damage in NIDDM rats." *Yakugaku Zasshi* 2006 May; 126(5): 365–371.

Wu SJ, Ng LT, Lin CC. "Antioxidant activities of some common ingredients of traditional Chinese medicine, *Angelica sinensis, Lycium barbarum* and *Poria cocos*." *Phytother Res* 2004 Dec; 18(12): 1008–1012.

Young G, Lawrence R and Schreuder M. *Discovery of the Ultimate Superfood.* Canandaigua, NY: Life Sciences Press, 2005.

Yu MS, Leung SK, Lai SW, et al. "Neuroprotective effects of anti-aging oriental medicine *Lycium barbarum* against beta-amyloid peptide neurotoxicity." *Exp Gerontol* 2005 Aug–Sep; 40(8-9): 716–727.

Zhang S. "Isolation and purification of *Lycium barbarum* polysaccharides and its antifatigue effect." *Wei Sheng Yan Jiu* 2000 Mar 30; 29(2): 115–117.

Zhao R, Li Q, Xiao B. "Effect of *Lycium barbarum* polysaccharide on the improvement of insulin resistance in NIDDM rats." *Yakugaku Zasshi* 2005 Dec; 125(12): 981–988.

Grapefruit

Baghurst K. "The Health Benefits of Citrus Fruits." Adelaide, CSIRO Health Sciences & Nutrition 2003 Dec. Available online at: www.australiancitrusgrowers.com/PDFs/projects/Health_Benefits_of_Citrus_Final_Report.pdf.

Cerda JJ, Normann SJ, Sullivan MP, et al. "Inhibition of atherosclerosis by dietary pectin in microswine with sustained hypercholesterolemia." *Circulation* 1994 Mar; 89(3): 1247–1253.

Dai Q, Borenstein AR, Wu Y, et al. "Fruit and vegetable juices and Alzheimer's disease: the Kame Project." *Am J Med* 2006 Sep; 119(9): 751–759.

Gao K, Henning SM, Niu Y, et al. "The citrus flavonoid naringenin stimulates DNA repair in prostate cancer cells." *J Nutr Biochem* 2006 Feb; 17(2): 89–95.

Gorinstein S, Caspi A, Libman I, et al. "Red grapefruit positively influences serum triglyceride level in patients suffering from coronary atherosclerosis: studies in vitro and in humans." *J Agric Food Chem* 2006 Mar 8; 54(5): 1887–1892.

Hahn-Obercyger M, Stark AH, Madar Z. "Grapefruit and oroblanco enhance hepatic detoxification enzymes in rats: possible role in protection against chemical carcinogenesis." *J Agric Food Chem* 2005 Mar 9; 53(5): 1828–1832.

Khaw KT, Bingham S, Welch A, et al. "Relation between plasma ascorbic acid and mortality in men and women in EPIC-Norfolk prospective study: a prospective population study." European Prospective Investigation into Cancer and Nutrition. *Lancet* 2001 Mar 3; 357(9257): 657–663.

Kurl S, Tuomainen TP, Laukkanen JA, et al. "Plasma vitamin C modifies the association between hypertension and risk of stroke." *Stroke* 2002 Jun; 33(6): 1568–1573.

Monroe KR, Murphy SP, Kolonel LN, et al. "Prospective study of grapefruit intake and risk of breast cancer in postmenopausal women: the Multiethnic Cohort Study." *Br J Cancer* 2007 Aug 6; 97(3): 440–445.

Morton JF. *Fruits of Warm Climates.* Miami, FL: Florida Flair Books, 1987.

Mullen W, Marks S, Crozier A. "Evaluation of phenolic compounds in commercial fruit juices and fruit drinks." *J Agric Food Chem* 2007 Apr 18; 55(8): 3148–3157.

Suzuki, KH, Sugie S, Murkami A, et al. "Citrus nobiletin inhibits azoxymethane-inducved rat colon carcinogenecis." Paper presented at the 228th ACS National Meeting, Aug 24, 2004, Philadelphia, PA.

Turner VJ, Leonardi T, Patil B, et al. "Grapefruit and its isolated bioactive compounds act as colon cancer chemo-protectants in rats." Paper presented at the 228th ACS National Meeting, Aug 24, 2004, Philadelphia, PA.

Mangoes

Ban JY, et al. "Neuroprotective properties of gallic acid from *Sanguisorbae radix* on amyloid beta protein (25–35)-induced toxicity in cultured rat cortical neurons." *Biol Pharm Bull* 2008 Jan; 31(1): 149–153.

Conca KR, Porter, WL, and Natick SD. "Antioxidant activity of mango puree and its component phenols." Soldier Center, U.S. Army Soldier and Biol. Chem. June 2002, Annual Meeting and Food Expo, Anaheim, CA.

"Hibiscus protocatechuic acid inhibits lipopolysaccharide-induced rat hepatic damage." *Archives of Toxicology* 2002 Apr 5. Available online at: www.springerlink.com/content/k8dvdtxra144t868.

Inoue M, et al. "Antioxidant, gallic acid, induces apoptosis in HL-60RG cells." *Biochem Biophys Res Commun* 1994 Oct 28; 204(2): 898–904.

Kim SH, Jun CD, Suk K, et al. "Gallic acid inhibits histamine release and pro-inflammatory cytokine production in mast cells." *Toxicol Sci* 2006; 91: 123–131.

Kroes BH, et al. "Anti-inflammatory activity of gallic acid." *Planta Med* 1992 Dec; 58(6): 499–504.

"Mangoes may protect against diabetes, high cholesterol." University of Queensland study presented at the Australian Health and Medical Research Congress, November 2006.

McCarty MF. "High-dose pyridoxine as an 'anti-stress' strategy." *Medical Hypotheses* 2000 May; 54(5): 803–807.

Raina K, et al. "Chemopreventive effects of oral gallic acid feeding on tumor growth and progression in TRAMP mice." *Mol Cancer Ther* 2008 May; 7(5): 1258–1267.

Sanae F, et al. "Potentiation of vasoconstrictor response and inhibition of endothelium-dependent vasorelaxation by gallic acid in rat aorta." *Planta Med* 2002 Aug; 68(8): 690–693.

"What is tannic acid?" *Phytochemicals*. Available online at: www.phytochemicals.info/phytochemicals/tannic-acid.php.

Yoshioka K, et al. "Induction of apoptosis by gallic acid in human stomach cancer KATO III and colon adenocarcinoma COLO 205 cell lines." *Oncol Rep* 2000 Nov-Dec; 7(6): 1221–1223.

Maple Syrup

Carl GF and Gallagher BB. "Manganese and epilepsy." In *Manganese in Health and Disease* by DL Klimis-Tavantzis (ed). Boca Raton, FL: CRC Press; 1994; 133–157.

Carpino A, Siciliano L, Petroni MF, et al. "Low seminal zinc bound to high molecular weight proteins in asthenozoospermic patients: evidence of increased sperm zinc content in oligoasthenozoospermic patients." *Hum Reprod* 1998; 13: 111–114.

Cerhan JR, Saag KG, Merlino LA, et al. "Antioxidant micronutrients and risk of rheumatoid arthritis in a cohort of older women." *Am J Epidemiol* 2003 Feb 15; 157(4): 345–354.

Chandra RK. "Micronutrients and immune functions." *Ann NY Acad Sci* 1990; 587: 9–16.

Constantinidis J. "Treatment of Alzheimer's disease by zinc compounds." *Drug Develop Res* 1992; 27: 1–14.

"Food for thought: studies probe role of minerals?in brain function." U.S. Dept of Agriculture 2005 Feb 9. Available online at: www.ars.usda.gov/is/AR/archive/oct01/brain1001.htm.

Goransson K, Liden S and Odsell L. "Oral zinc in acne vulgaris: a clinical and methodological study." *Acta Derm Venereol* 1978; 58: 443–448.

Keen CL, Zidenberg-Cherr S. "Manganese." In *Present Knowledge in Nutrition* (7th ed) by EE Ziegler EE and LJ Filer (eds). Washington, DC: ILSI Press, 1996; 334–343.

Kvist U, Kjellberg S, Bjorndahl L, et al. "Seminal fluid from men with agenesis of the Wolffian ducts: zinc-binding properties and effects on sperm chromatin stability." *Int J Androl* 1990; 13: 245–252.

Leach RM, Harris ED. "Manganese." In *Handbook of Nutritionally Essential Minerals* by BL O'Dell and RA Sunde (eds). New York, NY: Marcel Dekker, 1997; 335–355.

Muszynska A, Palka J, Gorodkiewicz E. "The mechanism of daunorubicin-induced inhibition of prolidase activity in human skin fibroblasts and its implication to impaired collagen biosynthesis." *Exp Toxicol Pathol* 2000; 52(2): 149–155.

Nowak G, Legutko B, et al. "Zinc treatment induces cortical brain-derived neurotrophic factor gene expression." *Eur J Pharmacol* 2004 May 10; 492(1): 57–59.

Ochi K, Ohashi T, Kinoshita H, et al. "The serum zinc level in patients with tinnitus and the effect of zinc treatment." *Nippon Jibiinkoka Gakkai Kaiho* 1997 Sep; 100(9): 915–919.

Shambaugh GE. "Zinc: the neglected nutrient." *Am J Otol* 1989 Mar; 10(2): 156–160.

Singh, et al, "Current zinc intake and risk of diabetes and coronary artery disease and factors associated with insulin resistance in rural and urban populations of north India." *J Amer Coll Nutr* 1998; 17: 564–570.

Stankovic H and Mikac-Devic D. "Zinc and copper in human semen." *Clin Chim Acta* 1976; 70: 123–126.

Strause L, Saltman P, Smith KT, et al. "Spinal bone loss in postmenopausal women supplemented with calcium and trace minerals." *J Nutr* 1994; 124(7): 1060–1064.

Tanaka Y. "A study of the role of zinc on the immune response and body metabolism: A contribution of trace elements." *Kobe J Med Sci* 1989 Dec; 35(5-6): 299–309.

Wada L and King JC. "Effect of low zinc intakes on basal metabolic rate, thyroid hormones and protein utilization in adult men." *J Nutr* 1986; 116: 1045–1053.

"Zinc could be key to eye disease." *BBC Health News* 2007 Mar 16. Available online at: news.bbc.co.uk/1/hi/health/6457427.stm.

Matcha

Adhami VM, Siddiqui IA, Ahmad N, et al. "Oral consumption of green tea polyphenols inhibits insulin-like growth factor-I-induced signaling in an autochthonous mouse model of prostate cancer." *Cancer Res* 2004 Dec 1; 64(23): 8715–8722.

Azam S, Hadi N, Khan NU, et al. "Pro-oxidant property of green tea polyphenols epicatechin and epigallocatechin-3-gallate: implications for anticancer properties." *Toxicol In Vitro* 2004 Oct; 18(5): 555–561.

Baek SJ, Kim JS, Jackson FR, et al. "Epicatechin gallate-induced expression of NAG-1 is associated with growth inhibition and apoptosis in colon cancer cells." *Carcinogenesis* 2004 Dec; 25(12): 2425–2432.

Bastianetto S, Yao ZX, Papadopoulos V, et al. "Neuroprotective effects of green and black teas and their catechin gallate esters against beta-amyloid-induced toxicity." *Eur J Neurosci* 2006 Jan; 23(1): 55–64.

Chen D, Daniel KG, Kuhn DJ, et al. "Green tea and tea polyphenols in cancer prevention." *Front Biosci* 2004 Sep 01; 9: 2618–2631.

Choi YB, Kim YI, Lee KS, et al. "Protective effect of epigallocatechin gallate on brain damage after transient middle cerebral artery occlusion in rats." *Brain Res* 2004 Sep 3; 1019(1-2): 47–54.

Coimbra S, Castro E, Rocha-Pereira P, et al. "The effect of green tea in oxidative stress." *Clin Nutr* 2006 Oct; 25(5): 790–796.

Devine A, Hodgson JM, Dick IM, et al. "Tea drinking is associated with benefits on bone density in older women." *Am J Clin Nutr* 2007 Oct; 86(4): 1243–1247.

Gates MA, Tworoger SS, Hecht JL, et al. "A prospective study of dietary flavonoid intake and incidence of epithelial ovarian cancer." *Int J Cancer* 2007 Nov 15; 121(10): 2225–2232.

Gouni-Berthold I and Sachinidis A. "Molecular mechanisms explaining the preventive effects of catechins on the development of proliferative diseases." *Curr Pharm Des* 2004; 10(11): 1261–1271.

"Green tea may protect the heart." *BBC Health News* 2005 Feb 26. Available online at: news.bbc. co.uk/go/pr/fr/-/1/hi/health/4298403.stm.

Haque AM, Hashimoto M, Katakura M, et al. "Long-term administration of green tea catechins improves spatial cognition learning ability in rats." *J Nutr* 2006 Apr; 136(4): 1043–1047.

Hussain T, Gupta S, Adhami VM, et al. "Green tea constituent epigallocatechin-3-gallate selectively inhibits COX-2 without affecting COX-1 expression in human prostate carcinoma cells." *Int J Cancer* 2005 Feb 10; 113(4): 660–669.

Ikeda I, Tsuda K, Suzuki Y, et al. "Tea catechins with agalloyl moiety suppress postprandial hypertriacylglycerolemia by delaying lymphatic transport of dietary fat in rats." *J Nutr* 2005 Feb; 135(2): 155–159.

Jian L, Lee AH, Binns CW. "Tea and lycopene protect against prostate cancer." *Asia Pac J Clin Nutr* 2007; 16 (Suppl 1): 453–457.

Kimura K, Ozeki M, Juneja LR, et al. "L-theanine reduces psychological and physiological stress responses." *Biol Psychol* 2007 Jan; 74(1): 39–45.

Koo MW and Cho CH. "Pharmacological effects of green tea on the gastrointestinal system." *Eur J Pharmacol* 2004 Oct 1; 500(1–3): 177–185.

Kurahashi N, Sasazuki S, Iwasaki M, et al. for the JPHC Study Group. "Green tea consumption and prostate cancer risk in japanese men: a prospective study." *Am J Epidemiol* 2008 Jan 1: 167(1): 71–77.

Kuriyama S, Hozawa A, Ohmori K, et al. "Green tea consumption and cognitive function: a cross-sectional study from the Tsurugaya Project." *Am J Clin Nutr* 2006 Feb; 83(2): 355–361.

Kuriyama S, Shimazu T, Ohmori K, et al. "Green tea consumption and mortality due to cardiovascular disease, cancer, and all causes in Japan: the Ohsaki study." *JAMA* 2006 Sep 13; 296(10): 1255–1265.

Liu YJ and Pan BS. "Inhibition of fish gill lipoxygenase and blood thinning effects of green tea extract." *J Agric Food Chem* 2004 Jul 28; 52(15): 4860–4864.

Murase T, Haramizu S, Shimotoyodome A, et al. "Green tea extract improves endurance capacity and increases muscle lipid oxidation in mice." *Am J Physiol Regul Integr Comp Physiol* 2005 Mar; 288(3): R708–R715.

Nagao T, Komine Y, Soga S, et al. "Ingestion of a tea rich in catechins leads to a reduction in body fat and malondialdehyde-modified LDL in men." *Am J Clin Nutr* 2005 Jan; 81(1): 122–129.

Ostrowska J, Luczaj W, Kasacka I, et al. "Green tea protects against ethanol-induced lipid peroxidation in rat organs." *Alcohol* 2004 Jan; 32(1): 25–32.

Reznichenko L, Amit T, Zheng H, et al. "Reduction of iron-regulated amyloid precursor protein and beta-amyloid peptide by (-)-epigallocatechin-3-gallate in cell cultures: implications for iron chelation in Alzheimer's disease." *J Neurochem* 2006 Apr; 97(2): 527–536.

Sakanaka S and Okada Y. "Inhibitory effects of green tea polyphenols on the production of a virulence factor of the periodontal-disease-causing anaerobic bacterium *Porphyromonas gingivalis*." *J Agric Food Chem* 2004 Mar 24; 52(6): 1688–1692.

Saleem M, Adhami VM, Siddiqui IA, et al. "Tea beverage in chemoprevention of Prostate cancer: a mini-review." *Nutr Cancer* 2003; 47(1): 13–23.

References

Sano J, Inami S, Seimiya K, et al. "Effects of green tea intake on the development of coronary artery disease." *Circ J* 2004 Jul; 68(7): 665–670.

Song JM, Lee KH, Seong BL. "Antiviral effect of catechins in green tea on influenza virus." *Antiviral Res* 2005 Nov; 68(2): 66–74.

Sun CL, Yuan JM, Koh WP, et al. "Green tea, black tea and breast cancer risk: a meta-analysis of epidemiological studies." *Carcinogenesis* 2006 Jul; 27(7):1310–1315.

Vinson JA, Teufel K, Wu N. "Green and black teas inhibit atherosclerosis by lipid, antioxidant, and fibrinolytic mechanisms." *J Agric Food Chem* 2004 Jun 2; 52(11): 3661–3665.

Weinreb O, Mandel S, Amit T, et al. "Neurological mechanisms of green tea polyphenols in Alzheimer's and Parkinson's diseases." *J Nutr Biochem* 2004 Sep; 15(9): 506–516.

Wu LY, Juan CC, Ho LT, et al. "Effect of green tea supplementation on insulin sensitivity in Sprague-Dawley rats." *J Agric Food Chem* 2004 Feb 11; 52(3): 643–648.

Wu LY, Juan CC, Hwang LS, et al. "Green tea supplementation ameliorates insulin resistance and increases glucose transporter IV content in a fructose-fed rat model." *Eur J Nutr* 2004 Apr; 43(2): 116–124.

Yang G, Shu XO, Li H, Chow WH, et al. "Prospective cohort study of green tea consumption and colorectal cancer risk in women." *Cancer Epidemiol Biomarkers Prev* 2007 Jun; 16(6): 1219–1223.

Yang YC, Lu FH, Wu JS, et al. "The protective effect of habitual tea consumption on hypertension." *Arch Intern Med* 2004 Jul 26; 164(14): 1534–1540.

Zhang M, Lee AH, Binns CW, et al. "Green tea consumption enhances survival of epithelial ovarian cancer." *Int J Cancer* 2004 Nov 10; 112(3): 465–469.

Zhang XH, Andreotti G, Gao YT, et al. "Tea drinking and the risk of biliary tract cancers and biliary stones: a population-based case-control study in Shanghai, China." *Int J Cancer* 2006 Jun 15; 118(12): 3089–3094.

Zheng G, Sayama K, Okubo T, et al. "Anti-obesity effects of three major components of green tea, catechins, caffeine and theanine, in mice." *In Vivo* 2004 Jan–Feb; 18(1): 55–62.

Millet

Anderson JW. "Whole grains and coronary Heart disease: the whole kernel of truth." *Am J Clin Nutr* 2004 Dec; 80(6): 1459–1460.

Bazzano LA, He J, Ogden LG, et al. "Dietary fiber intake and reduced risk of coronary heart disease in US men and women: the NHANES I Epidemiologic Follow-up Study." *Arch Intern Med* 2003 Sep 8; 163(16): 1897–1904.

Cade JE, Burley VJ, Greenwood DC. "Dietary fibre and risk of breast cancer in the UK Women's Cohort Study." *Int J Epidemiol* 2007 Apr; 36(2): 431–438.

Cashman KD. "Diet, nutrition, and bone health." *J Nutr* 2007 Nov; 137(Suppl 11): 2507S–2512S.

Coxam V. "Phyto-estrogens and bone health." *Proc Nutr Soc* 2008 May; 67(2): 184–195.

Delaney B, Nicolosi RJ, Wilson TA, et al. "Beta-glucan fractions from barley and oats are similarly antiatherogenic in hypercholesterolemic Syrian golden hamsters." *J Nutr* 2003 Feb; 133(2): 468–475.

Djoussé L and Gaziano JM. "Breakfast cereals and risk of heart failure in the Physicians' Health Study I." *Arch Intern Med* 2007 Oct 22; 167(19): 2080–2085.

Ensminger AH, Ensminger ME, Kondale JE, et al. *Foods & Nutrition Encyclopedia*. Clovis, CA: Pegus Press, 1983.

Erkkila AT, Herrington DM, Mozaffarian D, et al. "Cereal fiber and whole-grain intake are associated with reduced progression of coronary-artery atherosclerosis in postmenopausal women with coronary artery disease." *Am Heart J* 2005 Jul; 150(1): 94–101.

Goldberg B and Trivieri L. *Chronic Fatigue, Fibromyalgia & Lyme Disease* (2nd ed). Berkeley, CA: Celestial Arts, 2004.

Higdon J. "Thiamin." Micronutrient Information Center, Oregon State University Linus Pauling Institute, 2002. Available online at: lpi.oregonstate.edu/infocenter/vitamins/thiamin.

Jensen MK, Koh-Banerjee P, Hu FB, et al. "Intakes of whole grains, bran, and germ and the risk of coronary heart disease in men." *Am J Clin Nutr* 2004 Dec; 80(6): 1492–1499.

Johnsen NF, Hausner H, Olsen A, et al. "Intake of whole grains and vegetables determines the plasma enterolactone concentration of Danish women." *J Nutr* 2004 Oct; 134(10): 2691–2697.

Kligler B and Lee RA (eds). *Integrative Medicine.* New York, NY: McGraw-Hill, 2004.

Liu L, Zubik L, Collins FW, et al. "The antiatherogenic potential of oat phenolic compounds" *Atherosclerosis* 2004 Jul; 175(1): 39–49.

Marini H, Minutoli L, Polito F, et al. "Summaries for patients: effects of the phytoestrogen genistein on bone health in postmenopausal women." *Ann Intern Med* 2007 Jun 19; 146(12): 839–847.

Mayo Clinic. "Niacin (Vitamin B_3, Nicotinic Acid), Niacinamide." *MayoClinic.com* 2008 Jun 20. Available online at: www.mayoclinic.com/health/vitamin-B2/NS_patient-niacin.

Mayo Clinic. "Riboflavin (Vitamin B_2)." *MayoClinic.com* 2008 Jun 20. Available online at: www.mayoclinic.com/health/vitamin-B2/NS_patient-riboflavin.

Mayo Clinic. "Thiamine (Vitamin B_1)." *MayoClinic.com* 2008 Jun 20. Available online at: www.mayoclinic.com/health/vitamin-B2/NS_patient-thiamine.

Mayo Clinic. "Vitamin B_6." *MayoClinic.com* 2008 Jun 20. Available online at: www.mayoclinic.com/health/vitamin-B2/NS_patient-B6.

National Institute of Arthritis and Musculoskeletal and Skin Diseases. "Osteoporosis and menopause: phytoestrogens and bone health." NIAMS 2009 May. Available online at: www.niams.nih.gov/Health_Info/Bone/Osteoporosis/Menopause/default.asp.

Riemann D, et al. "The tryptophan depletion test: impact on sleep in primary insomnia." *Psychiatry Res* 2002; 109(2): 129–135.

Rosenstein DL, Elin, RJ, Hosseini JM, et al. "Magnesium measures across the menstrual cycle in premenstrual syndrome." *Biol Psychiatry* 1994 Apr 15; 35(8): 557–561.

Saltman PD and Strause LG. "The role of trace minerals in osteoporosis." *J Am Coll Nutr* 1993 Aug; 12(4): 384–389.

Suzuki R, Rylander-Rudqvist T, Ye W, et al. "Dietary fiber intake and risk of postmenopausal breast cancer defined by estrogen and progesterone receptor status—a prospective cohort study among Swedish women." *Int J Cancer* 2008 Jan 15; 122(2): 403–412.

Tabak C, Wijga AH, de Meer G, et al. "Diet and asthma in Dutch school children (ISAAC-2)." *Thorax* 2006 Dec; 61(12): 1048–1053.

Tsikitis VL, Albina JE, Reichner JS. "Beta-glucan affects leukocyte navigation in a complex chemotactic gradient." *Surgery* 2004 Aug; 136(2): 384–389.

van Dam RM, Hu FB, Rosenberg L, et al. "Dietary calcium and magnesium, major food sources, and risk of type 2 diabetes in U.S. Black women." *Diabetes Care* 2006 Oct; 29(10): 2238–2243.

Werbach MR. "Anxiety and the vitamin B complex." *Townsend Letter for Doctors and Patients* 2004 Oct. Available online at: www.townsendletter.com/Oct2004/nutinfluence1004.htm.

References

Miso

Baggott JE, et al. "Effect of miso (Japanese soybean paste) and NaCl on DMBA-induced rat mammary tumors." *Nutr Cancer* 1990; 14: 103–109.

Lawson W. "Be healthy with B$_{12}$." *Psychology Today* 2004 Feb 1. Available online at: www.psychologytoday.com/articles/pto-20040316-000003.html.

Sardesai V. *Introduction to Clinical Nutrition* (2nd ed). Boca Raton, FL: CRC Press, 2003.

Sorge C. "Combination of therapies offers help for IBS." *WebMD.com* 2004 Jul 8. Available online at: www.medicinenet.com/script/main/art.asp?articlekey=50294

Oats

Anderson JW, et al. "The oatmeal-cholesterol connection: 10 years later." 2008 *AJLM* 2008 Jan/Feb; 2: 51–57.

Anderson JW. "Whole grains and coronary Heart disease: the whole kernel of truth." *Am J Clin Nutr* 2004 Dec; 80(6): 1459–1460.

Bazzano LA, He J, Ogden LG, et al. "Dietary fiber intake and reduced risk of coronary heart disease in U.S. men and women: the NHANES I Epidemiologic Follow-up Study." *Arch Intern Med* 2003 Sep 8; 163(16): 1897–1904.

Cade JE, Burley VJ, Greenwood DC. "Dietary fibre and risk of breast cancer in the UK Women's Cohort Study." *Int J Epidemiol* 2007 Apr; 36)2): 431–438.

Cashman KD."Diet, nutrition, and bone health." *J Nutr* 2007 Nov; 137(11 Suppl): 2507S–2512S.

Chen CY, Milbury PE, Kwak HK, et al. "Avenanthramides phenolic acids from oats are bioavailable and act synergistically with vitamin C to enhance hamster and human LDL resistance to oxidation." *J Nutr* 2004 Jun; 134(6): 1459–1466.

Coxam V. "Phyto-oestrogens and bone health." *Proc Nutr Soc* 2008 May; 67(2): 184–195.

Delaney B, Nicolosi RJ, Wilson TA, et al. "Beta-glucan fractions from barley and oats are similarly antiatherogenic in hypercholesterolemic Syrian golden hamsters." *J Nutr* 2003 Feb; 133(2): 468–475.

Djoussé L and Gaziano JM. "Breakfast cereals and risk of heart failure in the Physicians' Health Study I." *Arch Intern Med* 2007 Oct 22; 167(19): 2080–2085.

Ensminger AH, Ensminger ME, Kondale JE, et al. *Foods & Nutrition Encyclopedia*. Clovis, CA: Pegus Press, 1983.

Erkkila AT, Herrington DM, Mozaffarian D, et al. "Cereal fiber and whole-grain intake are associated with reduced progression of coronary-artery atherosclerosis in postmenopausal women with coronary artery disease." *Am Heart J* 2005 Jul; 150(1): 94–101.

Goldberg B, Trivieri L. *Chronic Fatigue, Fibromyalgia & Lyme Disease* (2nd ed). Berkeley, CA: Celestial Arts, 2004.

Heaney RP, Nordin BE. "Calcium effects on phosphorus absorption: implications for the prevention and co-therapy of osteoporosis." *J Am Coll Nutr* 2002; 21(3): 239–244.

Higdon J. "Thiamin." Micronutrient Information Center, Oregon State University Linus Pauling Institute, 2002. Available online at: lpi.oregonstate.edu/infocenter/vitamins/thiamin.

Ishimi Y. "Prevention of osteoporosis by foods and dietary supplements: soybean isoflavone and bone metabolism." *Clin Calcium* 2006 Oct; 16(10): 1661–1667.

Jensen MK, Koh-Banerjee P, Hu FB, et al. "Intakes of whole grains, bran, and germ and the risk of coronary heart disease in men." *Am J Clin Nutr* 2004 Dec; 80(6): 1492–1499.

Johnsen NF, Hausner H, Olsen A, et al. "Intake of whole grains and vegetables determines the plasma enterolactone concentration of Danish women." *J Nutr* 2004 Oct; 134(10): 2691–2697.

Kligler B, Lee RA (eds). *Integrative Medicine*. New York, NY: McGraw-Hill, 2004.

Li W, Wei CV, White PJ, et al. "High-amylose corn exhibits better antioxidant activity than typical and waxy genotypes." *J Agric Food Chem* 2007 Jan 24; 55(2): 291–298.

Liu L, Zubik L, Collins FW, et al. "The antiatherogenic potential of oat phenolic compounds." *Atherosclerosis* 2004 Jul; 175(1): 39–49.

Marini H, Minutoli L, Polito F, et al. "Summaries for patients: effects of the phytoestrogen genistein on bone health in postmenopausal women." *Ann Intern Med* 2007 Jun 19; 146(12): 839–847.

Mayo Clinic. "Niacin (Vitamin B$_3$, Nicotinic Acid), Niacinamide." *MayoClinic.com* 2008 Jun 20. Available online at: www.mayoclinic.com/health/vitamin-B2/NS_patient-niacin.

Mayo Clinic. "Riboflavin (Vitamin B$_2$)." *MayoClinic.com* 2008 Jun 20. Available online at: www.mayoclinic.com/health/vitamin-B2/NS_patient-riboflavin.

Mayo Clinic. "Thiamine (Vitamin B$_1$)." *MayoClinic.com* 2008 Jun 20. Available online at: www.mayoclinic.com/health/vitamin-B2/NS_patient-thiamine.

Mayo Clinic. "Vitamin B$_6$." *MayoClinic.com* 2008 Jun 20. Available online at: www.mayoclinic.com/health/vitamin-B2/NS_patient-B6.

McCann's Irish Oatmeal. "Steel-cut oats." 2008. Available online at: www.mccanns.ie.

National Institute of Arthitis and Musculoskeletal and Skin Diseases. "Osteoporosis and menopause: phytoestrogens and bone health." NIAMS 2009 May. Available online at: www.niams.nih.gov/Health_Info/Bone/Osteoporosis/Menopause/default.asp.

Riemann D, et al. "The tryptophan depletion test: impact on sleep in primary insomnia." *Psychiatry Res* 2002; 109(2): 129–135.

Rosenstein DL, Elin, RJ, Hosseini JM, et al. "Magnesium measures across the menstrual cycle in premenstrual syndrome." *Biol Psychiatry* 1994 Apr 15; 35(8): 557–561.

Saltman PD and Strause LG. "The role of trace minerals in osteoporosis." *J Am Coll Nutr* 1993 Aug; 12(4): 384–389.

Suzuki R, Rylander-Rudqvist T, Ye W, et al. "Dietary fiber intake and risk of postmenopausal breast cancer defined by estrogen and progesterone receptor status—a prospective cohort study among Swedish women." *Int J Cancer* 2008 Jan 15; 122(2): 403–412.

Tabak C, Wijga AH, de Meer G, et al. "Diet and asthma in Dutch school children (ISAAC-2)." *Thorax* 2006 Dec; 61(12): 1048–1053.

Tsikitis VL, Albina JE, Reichner JS. "Beta-glucan affects leukocyte navigation in a complex chemotactic gradient." *Surgery* 2004 Aug; 136(2): 384–389.

van Dam RM, Hu FB, Rosenberg L, et al. "Dietary calcium and magnesium, major food sources, and risk of type 2 diabetes in U.S. Black women." *Diabetes Care* 2006 Oct; 29(10): 2238–2243.

Werbach MR. "Anxiety and the vitamin B complex." *Townsend Letter for Doctors and Patients* 2004 Oct. Available online at: www.townsendletter.com/Oct2004/nutinfluence1004.htm.

Whelan AM, Jurgens TM, Bowles SK. "Natural health products in the prevention and treatment of Osteoporosis: systematic review of randomized controlled trials." *Ann Pharmacother* 2006 May; 40(5): 836–849.

Wu J, Oka J, Ezaki J, et al. "Possible role of equol status in the effects of isoflavone on bone and fat mass in postmenopausal Japanese women: a double-blind, randomized, controlled trial." *Menopause* 2007 Sep–Oct; 14(5): 866–874.

Olives

Aguilera CM, Ramirez-Tortosa MC, Mesa MD, et al. "Protective effect of monounsaturated and polyunsaturated fatty acids on the development of cardiovascular disease." *Nutr Hosp* 2001 May–2001 Jun 30; 16(3): 78-91.

References

Bosetti C, Negri E, Franceschi S, et al. "Olive oil, seed oils and other added fats in relation to ovarian cancer." *Cancer Causes and Control* 2002 Jun; 13(5): 465–470.

Martinez-Dominguez E, de la Puerta R, Ruiz-Gutierrez V. "Protective effects upon experimental inflammation models of a polyphenol-supplemented virgin olive oil diet." *Inflamm Res* 2001 Feb; 50(2): 102–106.

Owen RW, Haubner R, Mier W, et al. "Isolation, structure elucidation and antioxidant potential of the major phenolic and flavonoid compounds in brined olive drupes." *Food Chem Toxicol* 2003 May; 41(5): 703–717.

Soltan MH and Jenkins DM. "Plasma copper and zinc concentrations and infertility." *International Journal of Obstetrics and Gynaecology* 2005 Aug 23; 90: 457–459.

Onions

92nd annual meeting of the American Association for Cancer Research (AACR) in New Orleans, March 26, 2001.

Boyer J, Brown D, Liu RH. "Uptake of quercetin 3-glucoside from whole onion and apple peel extracts by Caco-2 cell monolayers." *J Agric Food Chem* 2004 Nov 17; 52(23): 7172–7179.

Chen JH, Chen HI, Tsai SJ, et al. "Chronic consumption of raw but not boiled Welsh onion juice inhibits rat platelet function." *J Nutr* 2000; 130: 34–37.

Davis JM, Murphy EA, McClellan JL, et al. "Quercetin reduces susceptibility to influenza infection following stressful exercise." *Am J Physiol Regul Integr Comp Physiol* 2008 Jun; 295: R505–R509.

Galeone C, Pelucchi C, Levi F, et al. "Onion and garlic use and human cancer." *Am J Clin Nutr* 2006 Nov; 84(5): 1027–1032.

Hertog MGL, Feskens EJ, Hooman PC, et al. "Dietary antioxidant flavonoids and the risk of coronary heart disease: the Zutphen Elderly Study." *Lancet* 1993; 342: 1007–1011.

Huxley RR and Neil HAW. "The relation between dietary flavonol intake and coronary heart disease mortality: a meta-analysis of prospective cohort studies." *Eur J Clin Nutr* 2003; 57: 904–908.

Tjokroprawiro A, Pikir BS, Budhiarta AA, et al. "Metabolic effects of onion and green beans on diabetic patients." *Tohoku J Exp Med* 1983; 141(Suppl): 671–676.

Tolmunen S, Voutilainen J, Hintikka T. "Dietary folate and depressive symptoms are associated in middle-aged Finnish men." *J Nutr* 2003 Oct; 133(10): 3233–3236.

Vanderhoek J, Makheja A, Bailey J. "Inhibition of fatty acid lipoxygenases by onion and garlic oils: evidence for the mechanism by which these oils inhibit platelet aggregation." *Bioch Pharmacol* 1980; 29: 3169–3173.

Wetli HA, Brenneisen R, Tschudi I, et al. "A gamma-glutamyl peptide isolated from onion (*Allium cepa L.*) by bioassay-guided fractionation inhibits resorption activity of osteoclasts." *J Agric Food Chem* 2005 May 4; 53(9): 3408–3414.

Yang J, Meyers KJ, van der Heide J, et al. "Varietal differences in phenolic content and antioxidant and antiproliferative activities of onions." *J Agric Food Chem* 2004 Nov 3; 52(22): 6787–6793.

Oranges

American Chemical Society. "Mandarin oranges decrease liver cancer risk, atherosclerosis." 2006 Sept 11. Available online at: www.rxpg.com.

Guarnieri S, Riso P, et al. "Orange juice vs vitamin C: effect on hydrogen peroxide-induced DNA-damage in mononuclear blood cells." *Br J Nutr* 2007 Apr; 97(4): 639–643.

Honow R, Laube N, Schneider A, et al. "Influence of grapefruit-, orange- and apple-juice consumption on urinary variables and risk of crystallization." *Br J Nutr* 2003 Aug; 90(2): 295–300.

Khaw KT, Bingham S, Welch A, et al. "Relation between plasma ascorbic acid and mortality in men and women in EPIC-Norfolk prospective study: a prospective population study." *Lancet* 2001 Mar 3; 357(9257): 657–663.

Kurowska EM and Manthey JA. "Hypolipidemic effects and absorption of citrus polymethoxylated flavones in hamsters with diet-induced hypercholesterolemia." *J Agric Food Chem* 2004 May 19; 52(10): 2879–2886.

McIntosh M and Miller C. "A diet containing food rich in soluble and insoluble fiber improves glycemic control and reduces hyperlipidemia among patients with type 2 diabetes mellitus." *Nutr Rev* 2001 Feb; 59(2): 52–55.

Pereira MA and Ludwig DS. "Dietary fiber and body-weight regulation: observations and mechanisms." *Pediatr Clin North Am* 2001 Aug; 48(4): 969–980.

Pereira MA and Pins JJ. "Dietary fiber and cardiovascular disease: experimental and epidemiologic advances." *Curr Atheroscler Rep* 2000 Nov; 2(6): 494–502.

Simon JA, Hudes ES, Perez-Perez GI. "Relation of serum ascorbic acid to *Helicobacter pylori* serology in U.S. adults: the Third National Health and Nutrition Examination Survey." *J Am Coll Nutr* 2003 Aug; 22(4): 283–289.

Yuan JM, Stram DO, Arakawa K, et al. "Dietary cryptoxanthin and reduced risk of lung cancer: the Singapore Chinese Health Study." *Cancer Epidemiol Biomarkers Prev* 2003 Sep; 12(9): 890–898.

Zhao X, Yang Y, Song Z, et al. "Effect of superior fiber complex on insulin sensitivity index and blood lipids in non-insulin dependent diabetes mellitus rats." *Zhonghua Yu Fang Yi Xue Za Zhi* 2002 May; 36(3): 184–186.

CSIRO. "The health benefits of citrus fruits." CNN.com 2003 Dec. Available online at: www.cnn.com/2003/HEALTH/12/03/citrus.cancer.reut.

Pineapple

Akhtar NM, Naseer R, Farooqi AZ, et al. "Oral enzyme combination versus diclofenac in the treatment of osteoarthritis of the knee—a double-blind prospective randomized study." *Clin Rheumatol* 2004; 23: 410–415.

Balakrishnan V, Hareendran A, Nair CS. "Double-blind cross-over trial of an enzyme preparation in pancreatic steatorrhea." *J Assoc Physicians India* 1981; 29: 207–209.

Blonstein JL. "Control of swelling in boxing injuries." *Practitioner* 1969; 203: 206.

Chandler DS and Mynott TL. "Bromelain protects piglets from diarrhea caused by oral challenge with K88 positive enterotoxigenic *Escherichia coli*." *Gut* 1998; 43: 196–202.

Cho E, Seddon JM, Rosner B, et al. "Prospective study of intake of fruits, vegetables, vitamins, and carotenoids and risk of age-related maculopathy." *Arch Ophthalmol* 2004 Jun; 122(6): 883–892.

Cirelli MG. "Treatment of inflammation and edema with bromelain." *Delaware Med J* 1962; 34: 159–167.

Cohen A and Goldman J. "Bromelains therapy in rheumatoid arthritis." *Penn Med J* 1964; 67: 27–30.

Desser L, Rehberger A, Paukovits W. "Proteolytic enzymes and amylase induce cytokine production in peripheral blood mononuclear cells in vitro." *Cancer Biother* 1994; 9: 253–263.

Eckert K, Grabowska E, Stange R, et al. "Effects of oral bromelain administration on the impaired immunocytotoxicity of mononuclear cells from mammary tumor patients." *Oncol Rep* 1999; 6: 1191–1199.

Felton GE. "Fibrinolytic and antithrombotic action of bromelain may eliminate thrombosis in heart patients." *Med Hypotheses* 1980; 6(11): 1123–1133.

Kane S and Goldberg MJ. "Use of bromelain for mild ulcerative colitis [letter]." *Ann Intern Med* 2000; 132: 680.

Masson M. "Bromelain in blunt injuries of the locomotor system: a study of observed applications in general practice [in German; English abstract]. *Fortschr Med* 1995; 113: 303–306.

Masson M. "Bromelain in the treatment of blunt injuries to the musculoskeletal system: a case observation study by an orthopedic surgeon in private practice." *Fortschr Med* 1995; 113: 303–306.

References

Mori S, Ojima Y, Hirose T, et al. "The clinical effect of proteolytic enzyme-containing bromelain and trypsin on urinary tract infection evaluated by double blind method." *Acta Obstet Gynaecol Jpn* 1972; 19(3): 147–153.

Munzig E, Eckert K, Harrach T, et al. "Bromelain protease F9 reduces the CD44 mediated adhesions of human peripheral blood lymphocytes to human umbilical vein endothelial cells." *FEBS* Lett 1995; 351: 215–218.

Nieper HA. "Effect of bromelain on coronary heart disease and angina pectoris." *Acta Med Empirica* 1978; 5: 274–278.

Queensland Institute of Medical Research. "Pineapple stems that show anti-tumour activity." *Medical Research News* 2005 Jul 19. Available online at: www.qimr.edu.au.

Ryan RE. "A double-blind clinical evaluation of bromelains in the treatment of acute sinusitis." *Headache* 1967; 7: 13–17.

Schafer A and Adelman B. "Plasma inhibition of platelet function and of arachidonic acid metabolism." *J Clin Invest* 1985; 75: 456–461.

Seligman B. "Bromelain: an anti-inflammatory agent." *Angiology* 1962; 13: 508–510.

Seligman B. "Oral bromelains as adjuncts in the treatment of acute thrombophlebitis." *Angiology* 1969; 20: 22–26.

University of Maryland Medical Center. "Bromelain." UMMC 2009 Mar 14. Available online at: www.umm.edu/altmed/articles/bromelain-000289.htm.

Walker AF, Bundy R, Hicks SM, et al. "Bromelain reduces mild acute knee pain and improves well-being in a dose-dependent fashion in an open study of otherwise healthy adults." *Phytomedicine* 2002 Dec 9(8): 681–686.

Pomegranate

Aviram M, Rosenblat M, Gaitini D, et al. "Pomegranate juice consumption for 3 years by patients with carotid artery stenosis reduces common carotid intima-media thickness, blood pressure and LDL oxidation." *Clin Nutr* 2004 Jun; 23(3): 423–433.

Case Western Reserve University. "Pomegranate fruit shown to slow cartilage deterioration in osteoarthritis." *ScienceDaily.com* 2005 Sept 1. Available online at: www.sciencedaily.com/releases/2005/09/050901072114.htm.

Early Show, The. "Pomegranate ranked healthiest fruit juice." *CBSNews.com* 2008 Jul 5. Available online at: www.cbsnews.com/stories/2008/07/05/earlyshow/health/main4234811.shtml.

Forest CP, Padma-Nathan H, and Liker HR. "Efficacy and safety of pomegranate juice on improvement of erectile dysfunction in males with mild to moderate erectile dysfunction." *Int J Impo Res* 2007 Nov-Dec; 19(6): 564–567.

Khan N, Afaq F, Kweon MH. "Oral consumption of pomegranate fruit juice extract inhibits growth and progression of primary lung tumors in mice." *Can Res* 2007 Apr 1; 67(7): 3475–3482.

Lei F, Zhang XN, Wang W, et al. "Evidence of anti-obesity effects of the pomegranate leaf extract in high-fat diet induced obese mice." *Int J Obes* 2007 Jun; 31(6): 1023–1029.

Malik A. "Pomegranate fruit juice for chemoprevention and chemotherapy of prostate cancer." *Proc Natl Acad Sci* 2005; 102:14813–14818.

Malik A, Afaq F, Sarfaraz S, et al. "Pomegranate fruit juice for chemoprevention and chemotherapy of prostate cancer." *Proc Natl Acad Sci* 2005 Oct 11; 102(41): 14813–14818.

Mehta R, Lansky EP. "Breast cancer chemopreventive properties of pomegranate (*Punica granatum*) fruit extracts in mouse mammary organ culture." *Eur J Cancer Prev* 2004 Aug; 13(4): 345–348.

Mori-Okamoto J, Otawara-Hamamoto Y, Yamato H. "Pomegranate extract improves a depressive state and bone properties in menopausal syndrome model ovariectomized mice." *J Ethnopharmacol* 2004 May; 92(1): 93–101.

Murthy KN, Reddy VK, Veigas JM, et al. "Study on wound healing activity of *Punica granatum* peel." *J Med Food* 2004; 7(2): 256–259.

Sumner M, Elliot-Eller M, Weidner G, et al. "Effects of pomegranate juice consumption on myocardial perfusion in patients with coronary heart disease." *American Journal of Cardiology* 2005; 96(6): 810–814.

Turk G, Sönmez M, Aydın M, et al. "Effects of pomegranate juice consumption on sperm quality, spermatogenic cell density, antioxidant activity and testosterone level in male rats." *Clin Nutr* 2008 Apr 27(2): 289–296.

Yamasaki M, Kitagawa T, Koyanagi N, et al. "Dietary effect of pomegranate seed oil on immune function and lipid metabolism in mice." *Nutr* 2006 Jan; 22(1): 54–59.

Pumpkin

Ascherio A, Rimm EB, Hernan MA, et al. "Intake of potassium, magnesium, calcium, and fiber and risk of stroke among US men." *Circulation* 1998; 98(12): 1198–1204.

Barri YM and Wingo CS. "The effects of potassium depletion and supplementation on blood pressure: a clinical review." *Am J Med Sci* 1997; 314(1): 37–40.

"Clinical evidence for lutein and zeaxanthin in skin health, part 1: comparison of placebo, oral, topical and combined oral/topical xanthophylls treatments." Presented at Beyond Beauty Conference, Paris, September 13, 2006.

Curhan GC, Willett WC, Rimm EB, et al. "A prospective study of dietary calcium and other nutrients and the risk of symptomatic kidney stones." *N Engl J Med* 1993; 328(12): 833–838.

Curhan GC, Willett WC, Speizer FE, et al. "Comparison of dietary calcium with supplemental calcium and other nutrients as factors affecting the risk for kidney stones in women." *Ann Intern Med* 1997; 126(7): 497–504.

Grodstein F, Kang JH, Glynn RJ. "A randomized trial of beta carotene supplementation and cognitive function in men." *Arch Intern Med* 2007; 167(20): 2184–2190.

Holick CN, Michaud DS, Stolzenberg-Solomon R, et al. "Dietary carotenoids, serum beta-carotene, and retinol and risk of lung cancer in the alpha-tocopherol, beta-carotene cohort study." *Am J Epidemiol* 2002; 156(6): 536–547.

Hughes DA, Wright AJ, Finglas PM, et al. "The effect of beta-carotene supplementation on the immune function of blood monocytes from healthy male nonsmokers." *J Lab Clin Med* 1997; 129(3): 309–317.

Jian L, DU CJ, Lee AH, et al. "Do dietary lycopene and other carotenoids protect against prostate cancer?" *Int J Cancer* 2005 Mar 1; 113(6): 1010–1014.

Lyle BJ, et al. "Serum carotenoids and tocopherols and incidence of age-related nuclear cataract." *Am J Clin Nutr* 1999; 69: 272–277.

Malila N, Virtamo J, Virtanen M "The effect of a-Tocopherol and b-carotene supplementation on colorectal adenomas in middle-aged male smokers." *Cancer Epidemiol Biomarkers Prev* 1999 Jun 8; 489–493.

Mares-Perlman JA, et al. "Lutein and zeaxanthin in the diet and serum and their relation to age-related maculopathy in the Third National Health and Nutrition Examination Survey." *Am J Epidemiol* 2001; 153(5): 424–432.

New SA, Bolton-Smith C, Grubb DA, et al. "Nutritional influences on bone mineral density: a cross-sectional study in premenopausal women." *Am J Clin Nutr* 1997; 65(6): 1831–1839.

New SA, Robins SP, Campbell MK, et al. "Dietary influences on bone mass and bone metabolism: further evidence of a positive link between fruit and vegetable consumption and bone health?" *Am J Clin Nutr* 2000; 71(1): 142–151.

Santos MS, Gaziano JM, Leka LS, et al. "Beta-carotene-induced enhancement of natural killer cell activity in elderly men: an investigation of the role of cytokines." *Am J Clin Nutr* 1998; 68(1): 164–170.

Seddon JM, et al, "Dietary carotenoids, vitamins A, C, and E, and advanced age-related macular degeneration." *JAMA* 1994 Nov; 272(18): 1413–1420.

Sesso HD, Buring JE, Norkus EP, et al. "Plasma lycopene, other carotenoids, and retinol and the risk of cardiovascular disease in women." *Am J Clin Nutr* 2004; 79(1): 47–53.

References

Tucker KL, Hannan MT, Chen H, et al. "Potassium, magnesium, and fruit and vegetable intakes are associated with greater bone mineral density in elderly men and women." *Am J Clin Nutr* 1999; 69(4): 727–736.

van Poppel G, Spanhaak S, Ockhuizen T. "Effect of beta-carotene on immunological indexes in healthy male smokers." *Am J Clin Nutr* 1993; 57(3): 402–407.

Quinoa

Anderson JW. "Whole grains and coronary heart disease: the whole kernel of truth." *Am J Clin Nutr* 2004 Dec; 80(6): 1459–1460.

Cade JE, Burley VJ, Greenwood DC. "Dietary fibre and risk of breast cancer in the UK Women's Cohort Study." *Int J Epidemiol* 2007 Jan 24; 36(2): 413–438.

Jensen MK, Koh-Banerjee P, Hu FB, et al. "Intakes of whole grains, bran, and germ and the risk of coronary heart disease in men." *Am J Clin Nutr* 2004 Dec; 80(6): 1492–1499.

Liu RH. "New finding may be key to ending confusion over link between fiber, colon cancer." American Institute for Cancer Research. Press Release, Nov 4 2004.

Mauskop A and Altura BM. "Role of magnesium in the pathogenesis and treatment of migraines." *Clin Neurosci* 1998; 5(1): 24–27.

Mauskop A, et al. "Intravenous magnesium sulfate rapidly alleviates headaches of various types." *Headache* 1996; 36: 154–160.

Slattery ML, Curtin KP, Edward SL. "Plant foods, fiber, and rectal cancer." *AJCL* 2004 Feb; 79(2): 274–281.

Touyz RM. "Role of magnesium in the pathogenesis of hypertension." *Mol Aspects Med* 2003 Feb 6; 24(1–3): 107–136.

van Dam RM, Hu FB, Rosenberg L, et al. "Dietary calcium and magnesium, major food sources, and risk of type 2 diabetes in U.S. Black women." Diabetes Care 2006 Oct; 29(10): 2238–2243.

Red Wine

Baur JA, Pearson KJ, Price NL, et al. "Resveratrol improves health and survival of mice on a high-calorie diet." *Nature* 2006 Nov 16; 444: 337–342.

Cromie WJ. "Red wine protects against prostate cancer." *Harvard Men's Health Letter* 2007 Jun. Available online at: www.health.harvard.edu.

Daglia M, Papetti A, Grisoli P, et al. "Antibacterial activity of red and white wine against oral streptococc." *J Agric Food Chem* 2007; 55(13): 5038–5042.

Gonzales AM and Orlando RA. "Curcumin and resveratrol inhibit nuclear factor-kappaB-mediiated cytokine expression in adipocytes." *Nutr & Met* 2008; 5: 17.

Holian O, Wahid S, Atten MJ, et al. "Inhibition of gastric cancer cell proliferation by resveratrol: role of nitric oxide." *Am J Physiol Gastronintest Liver Physiol* 2002 May; 282(5): G809–G816.

Lu F, Zahid M, Wang C. "Resveratrol prevents estrogen-DNA adduct formation and neoplastic transformation in MCF-10F cells." *Cancer Prevention Research* 2008 Jul; 1: 135–145.

Marton KI. "Wine's antibacterial effect." *Journal Watch Cardiology* 1996 Mar 1: 15.

Moretro T, Daeschel MA. "Wine is bacterial to food-bourne pathogens." *J Food Sci* 2004 Nov/Dec 69(9): M251–M257.

Pearson KJ, Baur JA, and Lewis KN. "Resveratrol delays age-related deterioration and mimics transcriptional aspects of dietary restriction without extending lifespan." *Cell Metab* 2008 Aug 6; 8(2): 157–168.

"Resveratrol reduces number of fat cells." Endocrine Society's 90th Annual Meeting in San Francisco, June 16, 2008.

Thimothe J, Bonsi IA, Padilla-Zakour O. "Chemical characterization of red wine grape and pomace phenolic extracts and their biological activity against Streptococcus mutans." *J Agric Food Chem* 2007 55(13): 5038–5042.

Wang, J, Ho L, Zhao Z. "Moderate consumption of Cabernet savingnon attenuates Ab neuropathy in a mouse model of Alzheimer's disease." *FASEB Journal* 2006; 20: 2313–2320.

Weisse M, Eberly B, Person DA. "Wine as a digestive aid: comparative antimicrobial effects of bismuth salicylate and red and white wine." *BMJ* 1995 Dec 23; 311: 1657–1660.

Salmon

Bernard-Gallon DJ, Vissac-Sabatier C, Antoine-Vincent D, et al. "Differential effects of n-3 and n-6 polyunsaturated fatty acids on BRCA1 and BRCA2 gene expression in breast cell lines." *Br J Nutr* 2002 Apr; 87(4): 281–289.

Beydoun MA, Kaufman JS, Satia JA, et al. "Plasma n-3 fatty acids and the risk of cognitive decline in older adults: the Atherosclerosis Risk in Communities Study." *Am J Clin Nutr* 2007 Apr; 85(4): 1103–1111.

Calon F, Lim GP, Yang F, et al. "Docosahexaenoic acid protects from dendritic pathology in an Alzheimer's disease mouse model." *Neuron* 2004 Sep 2; 43(5): 633–645.

Chrysohoou C, Panagiotakos DB, Pitsavos C, et al. "Long-term fish consumption is associated with protection against arrhythmia in healthy persons in a Mediterranean region—the ATTICA study." *Am J Clin Nutr* 2007 May; 85(5): 1385–1391.

Chua B, Flood V, Rochtchina E, et al. "Dietary fatty acids and the 5-year incidence of age-related maculopathy." *Arch Ophthalmol* 2006 Jul; 124(7): 981–986.

Connor W. "Will the dietary intake of fish prevent atherosclerosis in diabetic women?" *Am J Clin Nutr* 2004 Sep; 80(3): 626–632.

Fritschi L, Ambrosini GL, Kliewer EV, et al. "Dietary fish intake and risk of leukaemia, multiple myeloma, and non-Hodgkin lymphoma." *Cancer Epidemiol Biomarkers Prev* 2004 Apr; 13(4): 532–537.

Ghose A, Fleming J, Harrison PR. "Selenium and signal transduction: roads to cell death and anti-tumor activity." *Biofactors* 2001; 14(1–4): 127–133.

He K, Song Y, Daviglus ML, et al. "Fish consumption and incidence of stroke: a meta-analysis of cohort studies." *Stroke* 2004 Jul; 35(7): 1538–1542.

Hedelin M, Chang ET, Wiklund F, et al. "Association of frequent consumption of fatty fish with prostate cancer risk is modified by COX-2 polymorphism." *Int J Cancer* 2007 Jan 15; 120(2): 398–405.

Iribarren C, Markovitz JH, Jacobs DR, et al. "Dietary intake of n-3, n-6 fatty acids and fish: relationship with hostility in young adults—the CARDIA study." *Eur J Clin Nutr* 2004 Jan; 58(1): 24–31

Kalmijn S, van Boxtel MP, Ocke M, et al. "Dietary intake of fatty aids and fish in relation to cognitive performance at middle age." *Neurology* 2004 Jan 27; 62(2): 275–280.

Lukiw WJ, Cui JG, Marcheselli VL, et al. "A role for docosahexaenoic acid-derived neuroprotectin D1 in neural cell survival and Alzheimer disease." *J Clin Invest* 2005 Oct; 115(10): 2774–2783.

Matute P. "Consumption of fish to allay obesity." Paper presented at the 6th Congress of the International Society for the Study of Fatty Acids and Lipids, Brighton, Great Britain, Dec 12, 2004.

Mazza M, Pomponi M, Janiri L, et al. "Omega-3 fatty acids and antioxidants in neurological and psychiatric diseases: an overview." *Prog Neuropsychopharmacol Biol Psychiatry* 2007 Jan 30; 31(1): 12–26.

Miljanovic B, Trivedi KA, Dana MR, et al. "Relation between dietary n-3 and n-6 fatty acids and clinically diagnosed dry eye syndrome in women." *Am J Clin Nutr* 2005 Oct; 82(4): 887–893.

Mozaffarian D, Psaty BM, Rimm EB, et al. "Fish intake and risk of incident atrial fibrillation." *Circulation* 2004 Jul 27; 110(4): 368–373.

References

Noaghiul S and Hibbeln JR. "Cross-national comparisons of seafood consumption and rates of bipolar disorders." *Am J Psychiatry* 2003 Dec; 160(12): 2222–2227.

Rose DP and Connolly JM. "Omega-3 fatty acids as cancer chemopreventive agents." *Pharmacol Ther* 1999 Sep; 83(3): 217–244.

Rose DP and Connolly JM. "Regulation of tumor angiogenesis by dietary fatty acids and eicosanoids." *Nutr Cancer* 2000; 37(2): 119–127.

Russell GR, Nader CJ, Patrick EJ. "Induction of DNA repair by some selenium compounds." *Cancer Lett* 1980 Jul; 10(1): 75–81.

Schaefer EJ, Bongard V, Beiser AS, et al. "Plasma phosphatidylcholine docosahexaenoic acid content and risk of dementia and Alzheimer disease: the Framingham Heart Study." *Arch Neurol* 2006 Nov; 63(11): 1545–1550.

Schwellenbach LJ, Olson KL, McConnell KJ, et al. "The triglyceride-lowering effects of a modest dose of docosahexaenoic acid alone versus in combination with low dose eicosapentaenoic acid in patients with coronary artery disease and elevated triglycerides" *J Am Coll Nutr* 2006 Dec; 25(6): 480–485.

Seddon JM, George S, and Rosner B. "Cigarette smoking, fish consumption, omega-3 fatty acid intake, and associations with age-related macular degeneration: the US Twin Study of age-related macular Degeneration." *Arch Ophthalmol* 2006 Jul; 124(7): 995–1001.

Serhan CN, Hong S, Gronert K, et al. "Resolvins: a family of bioactive products of omega-3 fatty acid transformation circuits initiated by aspirin treatment that counter proinflammation signals." *J Exp Med* 2002 Oct 21; 196(8): 1025–1037.

Steffen LM, Folsom AR, Cushman M, et al. "Greater fish, fruit, and vegetable intakes are related to lower incidence of venous thromboembolism: the longitudinal investigation of thromboembolism etiology." *Circulation* 2007 Jan 16; 115(2):188–195.

Stoll BA. "N-3 fatty acids and lipid peroxidation in breast cancer inhibition." *Br J Nutr* 2002 March; 87(3): 193–198.

Storey A, McArdle F, Friedmann PS, et al. "Eicosapentaenoic acid and docosahexaenoic acid reduce UVB- and TNF-alpha-induced IL-8 secretion in keratinocytes and UVB-induced IL-8 in fibroblasts." *J Invest Dermatol* 2005 Jan; 124(1): 248–255.

Sucher L and Moore L. Environmental Working Group (July 30, 2003).

Tabak C, Wijga AH, de Meer G, et al. "Diet and asthma in Dutch school children (ISAAC-2)." *Thorax* 2006 Dec; 61(12): 1048–1053.

Theodoratou E, McNeill G, Cetnarskyj R, et al. "Dietary fatty acids and colorectal cancer: a case-control study." *Am J Epidemiol* 2007 Jul 15; 166(2): 181–195.

Ueshima H, Stamler J, Elliott P, et al. "Food omega-3 fatty acid intake of individuals (total, linolenic acid, long-chain) and their blood pressure: INTERMAP Study." *Hypertension* 2007 Aug; 50(2): 313–319.

van Gelder BM, Tijhuis M, Kalmijn S, et al. "Fish consumption, n-3 fatty acids, and subsequent 5-y cognitive decline in elderly men: the Zutphen Elderly Study." *Am J Clin Nutr* 2007 Apr; 85(4): 1142–1147.

Vogt TM, Ziegler RG, Graubard BI, et al. "Serum selenium and risk of prostate cancer in U.S. blacks and whites." *Int J Cancer* 2003 Feb 20; 103(5): 664–670.

Wolk A, Larsson SC, Johansson JE, et al. "Long-term fatty fish consumption and renal cell carcinoma incidence in women." Swedish Mammography Cohort Study. *JAMA* 2006 Sep 20; 296(11): 1371–1176.

Wu M, Harvey KA, Ruzmetov N, et al. "Omega-3 polyunsaturated fatty acids attenuate breast cancer growth through activation of a neutral sphingomyelinase-mediated pathway." *Int J Cancer* 2005 Nov 10; 117(3): 340–348.

Sesame Seeds

Abbey LC. "Agoraphobia." *J Orthomol Psychiatry* 1982; 11: 243–259.

Bell IR, Edman JS, Morrow FD, et al. "B complex vitamin patterns in geriatric and young adult inpatients with major depression." *J Am Geriatr Soc* 1991 Mar; 39(3): 252–257.

Hyun T, Barrett-Connor E, and Milne D. "Zinc intakes and plasma concentrations in men with osteoporosis: the Rancho Bernardo Study." *Am J Clin Nutr* Sept. 2004: 80(3): 715–721.

Kita S, Matsumura Y, Morimoto S, et al. "Antihypertensive effect of sesamin, II: protection against two-kidney, one-clip renal hypertension and cardiovascular hypertrophy." *Biol Pharm Bull* 1995 Sep; 18(9): 1283–1285.

Matsumura Y, Kita S, Morimoto S, et al. "Antihypertensive effect of sesamin, I: protection against deoxycorticosterone acetate-salt-induced hypertension and cardiovascular hypertrophy." *Biol Pharm Bull* 1995 Jul; 18(7): 1016–1019.

Nakai M, Harada M, Nakahara K, et al. "Novel antioxidative metabolites in rat liver with ingested sesamin." *J Agric Food Chem* 2003 Mar 12; 51(6): 1666–1670.

Ogawa H, Sasagawa S, Murakami T, et al. "Sesame lignans modulate cholesterol metabolism in the stroke-prone spontaneously hypertensive rat." *Clin Exp Pharmacol Physiol* 1995 Dec; 22 (Suppl 1): S310–S312.

Phillips KM, Ruggio DM, Ashraf-Khorassani M. "Phytosterol composition of nuts and seeds commonly consumed in the United States." *J Agric Food Chem* 2005 Nov 30; 53(24): 9436–9445.

Sirato-Yasumoto S, Katsuta M, Okuyama Y, et al. "Effect of sesame seeds rich in sesamin and sesamolin on fatty acid oxidation in rat liver." *J Agric Food Chem* 2001 May; 49(5): 2647–2651.

Thys-Jacobs S, Starkey P, Bernstein D, et al. "Calcium carbonate and the premenstrual syndrome: effects on premenstrual and menstrual symptoms." Premenstrual syndrome study group. *Am J Obstet Gynecol* 1998; 179(2): 444–452.

Shiitake Mushrooms

American Chemical Society. Research presented at the American Chemical Society meeting in Washington, DC, 2005.

Cochran KW, et al. "Botanical sources of influenza inhibitors." *Antimicrobial Agents and Chemotherapy* 1966: 515–520.

Fukushima M, Ohashi T, Fujiwara Y, et al. "Cholesterol-lowering effects of maitake (*Grifola frondosa*) fiber, shiitake (*Lentinus edodes*) fiber, and enokitake (*Flammulina velutipes*) fiber in rats." *Exp Biol Med* 2001 Sep; 226(8): 758–765.

Gordon M, Bihari B, Goosby E, et al. "A placebo-controlled trial of the immune modulator, lentinan, in HIV-positive patients: a phase I/II trial." *J Med* 1998; 29(5–6): 305–330.

Harada T, et al. "Therapeutic effect of LEM (extract of cultured *Lentinus edodes mycelia*) against HBeAg-positive chronic hepatitis B." (Abstract 719) *Gastroenterol Intl* 1988; 1 (Suppl 1).

Hayakawa M, Kuzuya F. "Studies on platelet aggregation and cortinellus shiitake." *Nippon Ronen Igakkai Zasshi* 1985 Mar; 22(2): 151–159.

Nanba H and Kuroda H. "Antitumor mechanisms of orally administered shiitake fruit bodies." *Chem Pharm Bull* (Tokyo) 1987 Jun; 35(6): 2459–2464.

Nanba H, Mori K, Toyomasu T, et al. "Antitumor action of shiitake (*Lentinus edodes*) fruit bodies orally administered to mice." *Chem Pharm Bull* (Tokyo) 1987 Jun; 35(6): 2453–2458.

Ng ML and Yap AT. "Inhibition of human colon carcinoma development by lentinan from shiitake mushrooms (*Lentinus edodes*)." *J Altern Complement Med* 2002 Oct; 8(5): 581–589.

References

Ogawa K, Wantanabe T, Katsube T, et al. "Study on intratumor administration of lentinan—primary changes in cancerous tissues." *Gan To Kagaku Ryoho* 1994 Sep; 21 [Article in Japanese; abstract in English].

Papa CM. "Topical erythromycin and zinc for acne." *J Am Acad Dermatol* 1991 Feb; 24(2 Pt 1): 318–319.

Shouji N, et al. "Anticaries effect of a component from shiitake (an edible mushroom)." *Carie Res* 2000 Feb; 34(1): 94–98.

Suzuki M, Iwashiro M, Takatsuki F, et al. "Reconstitution of anti-tumor effects of lentinan in nude mice: roles of delayed-type hypersensitivity reaction triggered by CD4 positive T cell clone in the infiltration of." *Jpn J Cancer Res* 1994; 85(4): 409–417.

Takazawa H, Tajima F, and Miyashita C. "An antifungal compound from 'shiitake' (*Lentinus edodes*)." *Yakugaku Zasshi* 1982 May; 102(5): 489–491.

Takehara M, Mori K, Kuida K, et al. "Antitumor effect of virus-like particles from *Lentinus edodes* (shiitake) on Ehrlich ascites carcinoma in mice." *Arch Virol* 1981; 68(3–4): 297–301.

Takehara M, Toyomasu T, Mori K, et al. "Isolation and antiviral activities of the double-stranded RNA from *Lentinus edodes* (shiitake)." *Kobe J Med Sci* 1984 Aug; 30(3–4): 25–34.

Spinach

Albanes D. "The effect of a-tocopherol and b-carotene supplementation on colorectal adenomas in middle-aged male smokers." *Cancer Epidemiology Biomarkers & Prevention* 1999 Jun; 8: 489–493.

American Society for Nutritional Sciences. *J Nutr* 2003 Nov; 133: 3598–3602.

Comstock GW, Burke AE, Hoffman SC, et al. "Serum concentrations of a-tocopherol, b-carotene, and retinol preceding the diagnosis of rheumatoid arthritis and systemic lupus erythematosus." *Ann Rheum Dis* 1997 May; 56: 323–325.

Ford ES. "Serum magnesium and ischaemia heart disease: findings from a national sample of US adults." *Int J Epidemiol* 1999 Aug; 28(4): 645–651.

Gates MA, Tworoger SS, Hecht JL, et al. "A prospective study of dietary flavonoid intake and incidence of epithelial ovarian cancer." *Int J Cancer* 2007 Nov 15; 121(10): 2225–2232.

Hosseinzadeh, et al. "Antidepressant effect of kaempferol, a constituent of saffron (*Crocus sativus*) petal, in mice and rats." *Pharmacologyonline* 2007; 2: 367–370.

Jian L, Du CJ, Lee AH, et al. "Do dietary lycopene and other carotenoids protect against prostate cancer?" *Int J Cancer* 2005 Mar 1: 113(6): 1010–1014.

Joseph JA, Shukitt-Hale B, Denisova NA, et al. "Long-term dietary strawberry, spinach, or vitamin E supplementation retards the onset of age-related neuronal signal-transduction and cognitive behavioral deficits." *J Neurosci* 1998 Oct 1; 18(19): 8047–8055.

Joseph JA, Shukitt-Hale B, Denisova NA, et al. "Reversals of age-related declines in neuronal signal transduction, cognitive, and motor behavioral deficits with blueberry, spinach, or strawberry dietary supplementation." *J Neurosci* 1999 Sep 15; 19(18): 8114–8121.

Longnecker MP, Newcomb PA, Mittendorf R, et al. "Intake of carrots, spinach, and supplements containing vitamin A in relation to risk of breast cancer." *Cancer Epidemiol Biomarkers Prev* 1997 Nov; 6(11): 887–892.

Manach C, Scalbert A, Morand C, et al. "Polphenols: food sources and bioavailability." *Am J Clin Nutr* 2004 May; 79(5): 727–747.

Mauskop A and Altura BM. "Role of magnesium in the pathogenesis and treatment of migraines." *Clin Neurosci* 1998; 5(1): 24–27.

Morris MC, Evans DA, Tangney CC, et al. "Associations of vegetable and fruit consumption with age-related cognitive change." *Neurology* 2006 Oct 24; 67(8): 1370–1376.

National Academy of Sciences. *Proc Nat Acad Sci,* Nov. 27, 2001.

Nöthlings U, Murphy SP, Wilkens LR, et al. "Flavonols and pancreatic cancer risk," *Am J Epidemiol* 2007; 166(8): 924–931.

Seddon JM, Ajani UA, Sperduto RD, et al. "Dietary carotenoids, vitamins A, C, and E, and advanced age-related macular degeneration." Eye Disease Case-Control Study Group. *JAMA* 1994 Nov 9; 272(18): 1413–1420.

Tucker KT, Hannan MT, Chen H, et al. "Potassium, magnesium, and fruit and vegetable intakes are associated with greater bone density in elderly men and women." *Am J Clin Nutr* 1999; 69: 727–736.

Wang, et al. "Vitamin B_{12} and folate in relation to the development of Alzheimer's disease." *Neurology* 2001 May 8; 56: 1188–1194.

Watson RR, ed. *Functional Foods & Nutraceuticals in Cancer Prevention.* New York, NY: John Wiley & Sons, 2003.

Yang Y, Marczak ED, Yokoo M, et al. "Isolation and antihypertensive effect of angiotensin I-converting enzyme (ACE) inhibitory peptides from spinach Rubisco." *J Agric Food Chem* 2003 Aug 13; 51(17): 4897–4902.

Zhang X, Chinkes D, Wolfe R. "Leucine supplementation has an anabolic effect on proteins in rabbit skin wound and muscle." *J Nutr* 2004 Dec; 134: 3313–3318.

Strawberries

Cho E, Seddon JM, Rosner B, et al. "Prospective study of intake of fruits, vegetables, vitamins, and carotenoids and risk of age-related maculopathy." *Arch Ophthalmol* 2004 Jun; 122(6): 883–892.

Joseph JA, Shukitt-Hale B, Denisova NA, et al. "Long-term dietary strawberry, spinach or vitamin E supplementation retards the onset of age-related neuronal signal-transduction and cognitive behavioral deficits." *J Neurosci* 1998 Oct 1; 18(19): 8047–8055.

Joseph JA, Shukitt-Hale B, Denisova NA, et al. "Reversals of age-related declines in neuronal signal transduction, cognitive, and motor behavioral deficits with blueberry, spinach, or strawberry dietary supplementation." *J Neurosci* 1999 Sep 15; 19(18): 8114–8121.

Kahkonen MP, Hopia AI, Heinonen M. "Berry phenolics and their antioxidant activity." *J Agric Food Chem* 2001 Aug; 49(8): 4076–4082.

Kalt W, Forney CF, Martin A, et al. "Antioxidant capacity, vitamin C, phenolics, and anthocyanins after fresh storage of small fruits." *J Agric Food Chem* 1999 Nov; 47(11): 4638–4644.

Meyers KJ, Watkins CB, Pritts MP, et al. "Antioxidant and antiproliferative activities of strawberries." *J Agric Food Chem* 2003 Nov 5; 51(23): 6887–6892.

Pattison DJ, Silman AJ, Goodson NJ, et al. "Vitamin C and the risk of developing inflammatory polyarthritis: prospective nested case-control study." *Ann Rheum Dis* 2004 Jul; 63(7): 843–847.

Zhang W, Jin MF, Yu XJ, et al. "Enhanced anthocyanin production by repeated-batch culture of strawberry cells with medium shift." *Appl Microbiol Biotechnol* 2001 Mar; 55(2): 164–169.

Sweet Potatoes

Cook N, Stampfer MJ, Ma J, et al. "Beta-carotene supplementation for patients with low baseline levels and decreased risks of total and prostate carcinoma." *Cancer* 1999; 86: 1783–1792.

DiGiovanna JJ. "Retinoid chemoprevention in patients at high risk for skin cancer." *Med Pediatr Oncol* 2001; 36: 564–567.

Gaziano JM, Manson JE, Branch LG, et al. "A prospective study of consumption of carotenoids in fruits and vegetables and decreased cardiovascular mortality in the elderly." *Ann Epidemiol* 1995; 5: 255–260.

References

Grodstein F, Kang JH, Glynn RJ, et al. "A randomized trial of beta-carotene supplementation and cognitive function in men." *Archives of Internal Medicine* 2007 Nov 12; 167(20): 2184–2190.

Hankinson SE, Stampfer MJ, Seddon JM, et al. "Nutrient intake and cataract extraction in women: a prospective study." *BMJ* 1992; 305(6849): 335–339.

Ruano-Ravina A, Figueiras A, Barros-Dios JM. "Diet and lung cancer: a new approach." *Eur J Cancer Prev* 2000; 9: 395–400.

Wertz K, Seifert N, Hunziker PB, et al. "Beta-carotene inhibits UVA-induced matrix metalloprotease 1 and 10 expression in keratinocytes by a singlet oxygen-dependent mechanism." *Free Radic Biol Med* 2004; 37: 654–670.

Ylonen K, Alfthan G, Groop L, et al. "Dietary intakes and plasma concentrations of carotenoids and tocopherols in relation to glucose metabolism in subjects at high risk of type 2 diabetes: the Botnia Dietary Study." *Am J Clin Nutr* 2003 Jun; 77(6): 1434–1441.

Zhang S, Hunger DJ, Forman MR, et al. "Dietary carotenoids and vitamins A, C, and E and risk of breast cancer." *J Natl Cancer Inst* 1999; 91: 547–556.

Tomatoes

All India Institute of Medical Sciences. "Fruit fights infertility." *BBC News Online* 2001 Mar 12. Available online at: news.bbc.co.uk/2/hi/health/1211475.stm.

Goyal A, Chopra M, Lwaleed BA, et al. "Effects of dietary lycopene on human seminal plasma." *BJU Int* 2007 Jun; 99(6): 1456–1460.

Kavanaugh CJ, Trumbo PR, Ellwood KC. "The U.S. Food and Drug Administration's evidence-based review for qualified health claims: tomatoes, lycopene, and cancer." *J Natl Cancer Inst* 2007 Jul 18; 99(14): 1074–1085.

Palan P and Naz R. "Changes in various antioxidant levels in human seminal plasma related to immunoinfertility." *Arch Androl* 1996 Mar–Apr; 36(2): 139–143.

University of Illinois at Urbana-Champaign. "Lycopene's anti-cancer effect linked to other tomato components." *ScienceDaily.com* 2003 Nov 5. Available online at: www.sciencedaily.com/releases/2003/11/031105064728.htm.

Tuna

Benito-Leon J and Porta-Etessam J. "Shaky-leg syndrome and vitamin B_{12} deficiency." *N Engl J Med* 2000; 342: 981.

"Cigarette smoking, fish consumption, omega-3 fatty acid intake, and associations with age-related macular degeneration." *Arch Ophthalmol* 2006 Jul; 124(7): 995–1001.

Connor WE and Connor SL. "The importance of fish and docosahexaenoic acid in Alzheimer disease." *Am J Clin Nutr* 2007 Apr; 85(4): 929–930.

Diplock AT. "Selenium, antioxidant nutritions, and human diseases." *Biol Trac Elem Res* 1992; 33: 155–156.

Erkkila A, Lichtenstein A, Mozaffarian D, et al. "Fish intake is associated with a reduced progression of coronary artery atherosclerosis in postmenopausal women with coronary artery disease." *Am J Clin Nutr* 2004 Sept; 80(3): 626–632.

Fritschi L, Ambrosini GL, Kliewer EV, et al. "Dietary fish intake and risk of leukemia, multiple myeloma, and non-Hodgkin lymphoma." *Cancer Epidemiology Biomarkers & Prevention* 2004 Apr; 13(4): 532–537.

Galarraga B, Ho M, Youssef HM, et al. "Cod liver oil (n-3 fatty acids) as an non-steroidal anti-inflammatory drug sparing agent in rheumatoid arthritis." *Rheumatol* 2008 Mar; 47(5): 665–669.

Grases G, Perez-Castello JA, Sanchis P, et al. "Anxiety and stress among science students: study of calcium and magnesium alterations." *Magnes Res* 2006 Jun; 19(2): 102–106.

He K, Song Y, Daviglus ML, et al. "Fish consumption and incidence of stroke." *Stroke,* 2004; 35: 1538.

Holguin F, Tellez-Rojo MM, Lazo M, et al. "Cardiac autonomic changes associated with fish oil vs soy oil supplementation in the elderly." *Chest* 2005 Apr; 127(4): 1102–1107.

Iribarren C, Markovitz JH, Jacobs DR, et al. "Dietary intake of n-3, n-6 fatty acids and fish: relationship with hostility in young adults-the CARDIA study." *Eur J Clin Nutr* 2004 Jan; 58(1): 24–31.

Iso H, Kobayashi M, Ishihara J, et al. "Intake of fish and n3-fatty acids and risk of coronary heart disease among Japanese." *Circulation* 2006 Jan 17; 113(2): 195–202.

Koch C, Dölle S, Metzger M, et al. "Docosahexaenoic acid (DHA) supplementation in atopic eczema: a randomized, double-blind, controlled trial." *Br J Dermatol* 2008 Apr; 158(4): 786–792.

Maes M and Smith RS. "Fatty acids, cytokines, and major depression." *Biol Psychiatry,* 1998; 43: 313–314.

Matute P. "Consumption of fish to allay obesity." Paper presented at the 6th Congress of the International Society for the Study of Fatty Acids and Lipids, Brighton, Great Britain, December 12, 2004.

McCaddon A and Kelly C. "Familial Alzheimer's disease and vitamin B_{12} deficiency." *Age and Ageing* 1994 Jul; 23: 334–337.

Miljanovic B, Trivedi KA, Dana MR, et al. "Relation between dietary n-3 and n-6 fatty acids and clinically diagnosed dry eye syndrome in women." *Am J Clin Nutr* 2005 Oct; 82(4): 887–893.

Mozaffarian D, Psaty BM, Rimm E, et al. "Fish intake and risk of incident of arterial fibrillation." *Circulation* 2004 Jul 24; 110(4): 368–373.

National Osteoporosis Foundation. Fifth International Symposium, March 9, 2002.

Rhodes LE, Shahbakhti H, Azurdia RM. "Effect of eicosapentaenoic acid, an omega-3 polyunsaturated fatty acid, on UVR-related cancer risk in humans." *Carcinogenesis* 2003 May; 24(5): 919–925.

Schwellenbach, LJ. "The triglyceride-lowering effects of a modest dose of docosahexaenoic acid alone versus in combination with low dose eicosapentaenoic acid in patients with coronary artery disease and elevated triglycerides." *J Am Coll Nutr* 2006 25(6): 480–485.

Steenhuysen J. "Omega-3 fatty acids protect against diabetes: study." *Reuters online* 2007 Sept 25. Available online at: www.reuters.com/article/healthNews/idUSN2540481120070925?feedType=RSS&feedName=healthNews&pageNumber=2&virtualBrandChannel=0.

Steffen LM, Jacobs DR, Stevens J, et al. "Heightened risk of deep-vein thrombosis." *Circulation* 2001; 104: 2442–2446.

Storey A. "Eicosapentaenoic acid and docosahexaenoic acid reduce UVB- and TNF-alpha-induced IL-8 secretion in keratinocytes and UVB-induced IL-8 in fibroblasts." *J Invest Dermatol* 2005 Jan; 124(1): 248–255.

Su K, Huang S, Chiu T, et al. "Omega-3 fatty acids for major depressive disorder during pregnancy: results from a randomized, double-blind, placebo-controlled trial." *J Clin Psychiatry,* 2008 Apr; 69(4): 644–651.

Tabak C, Wijga AH, and Smit HA. "Diet and asthma in Dutch schoolchildren." *Thorax* 2006; 61: 1048–1053.

Theodoratou E, McNeill G, et al. "Dietary fatty acids and colorectal cancer: a case control study." *Am J Epidemiol* 2007 Jul 15; 166(2): 181–195.

USDA/ARS. "Fight Osteoporosis: bone up on B_{12}." *ScienceDaily.com* 2005 Apr 23. Available online at www.sciencedaily.com/releases/2005/04/050421235233.htm.

Vogt TM, Ziegler RG, Graubard BI, et al. "Serum selenium and risk of prostate cancer in U.S. blacks and whites." *Int J Cancer* 2003 Feb 20; 103(5): 664–670.

Werbach MR. "Nutritional strategies for treating chronic fatigue syndrome." *Altern Med Rev* 2000; 5: 93–108.

Wolk A, Larsson SC, Johansson JE, et al. "Long-term fatty fish consumption and renal cell caranoma incidence in women." Swedish Mammography Cohort Study. *JAMA* 2006; 296: 1371–1376.

References

Wu M, Harvey KA, Ruzmetov N, et al. "Omega-3 polyunsaturated fatty acids attenuate breast cancer growth through activation of a neural sphingomyelinase-mediated pathway." *Int J Cancer* 2005 Nov 10; 117(3): 340–348.

Turmeric

Abbey M, Noakes M, Belling GB, et al. "Partial replacement of saturated fatty acids with almonds or walnuts lowers total plasma cholesterol and low-density-lipoprotein cholesterol." *Am J Clin Nutr* 1994 May; 59(5): 995–999.

Aggarwal B. Paper presented at the U.S. Defense Department's "Era of Hope" Breast Cancer Research Program meeting in Philadelphia, PA, October 5, 2005. Reported in NUTRAingredients.com/Europe. "Turmeric slows breast cancer spread in mice."

Asai A, Nakagawa K, Miyazawa T. "Antioxidative effects of turmeric, rosemary and capsicum extracts on membrane phospholipid peroxidation and liver lipid metabolism in mice." *Biosci Biotechnol Biochem* 1999 Dec; 63(12): 2118–2122.

Balasubramanian K. "Molecular orbital basis for yellow curry spice curcumin's prevention of Alzheimer's disease." *J Agric Food Chem* 2006; 54 (10): 3512–3520.

Calabrese V, Butterfield DA, Stella AM. "Nutritional antioxidants and the heme oxygenase pathway of stress tolerance: novel targets for neuroprotection in Alzheimer's disease." *Ital J Biochem* 2003 Dec; 52(4): 177–181.

Cruz-Correa M, Shoskes DA, Sanchez P, et al. "Combination treatment with curcumin and quercetin of adenomas in familial adenomatous polyposis." *Clin Gastroenterol Hepatol* 2006 Aug; 4(8): 1035–1038.

Deshpande UR, Gadre SG, Raste AS, et al. "Protective effect of turmeric (*Curcuma longa L.*) extract on carbon tetrachloride-induced liver damage in rats." *Indian J Exp Biol* 1998 Jun; 36(6): 573–577.

Dorai T, Cao YC, Dorai B, et al. "Therapeutic potential of curcumin in human prostate cancer, III: curcumin inhibits proliferation, induces apoptosis, and inhibits angiogenesis of LNCaP prostate cancer cells in vivo." *Prostate* 2001 Jun 1; 47(4): 293–303.

Egan ME, Pearson M, Weiner SA, et al. "Curcumin, a major constituent of turmeric, corrects cystic fibrosis defects." *Science* 2004 Apr 23; 304(5670): 600–602.

Fiala M, Liu PT, Espinosa-Jeffrey A, et al. "Innate immunity and transcription of MGAT-III and Toll-like receptors in Alzheimer's disease pateints are improved by bisdemethoxycurcumin." *Proc Natl Acad Sci USA* 2007 Jul 31; 104(31): 12849–12854.

Funk JL, Frye JB, Oyarzo JN, et al. "Efficacy and mechanism of action of turmeric supplements in the treatment of experimental arthritis." *Arthritis Rheum* 2006 Nov; 54(11): 3452–3464.

Kang BY, Chung SW, Chung W, et al. "Inhibition of interleukin-12 production in lipopolysaccharide-activated macrophages by curcumin." *Eur J Pharmacol* 1999 Nov 19; 384(2–3): 191–195.

Kang BY, Song YJ, Kim KM, et al. "Curcumin inhibits Th1 cytokine profile in CD4+ T cells by suppressing interleukin-12 production in macrophages." *Br J Pharmacol* 1999 Sept; 128(2): 380–384.

Karunagaran D, Rashmi R, Kumar TR. "Induction of apoptosis by curcumin and its implications for cancer therapy." *Curr Cancer Drug Targets* 2005 Mar; 5(2): 117–129.

Kawamori T, Lubet R, Steele VE, et al. "Chemopreventive effect of curcumin: a naturally occurring anti-inflammatory agent, during the promotion/progression stages of colon cancer." *Cancer Res* 1999; 59: 597–601.

Khor TO, Keum YS, Lin W, et al. "Combined inhibitory effects of curcumin and phenethyl isothiocyanate on the growth of human PC-3 prostate xenografts in immunodeficient mice." *Can Res* 2006 Jan; 66(2): 613–621.

Kurd SK, Smith N, VanVoorhees A, et al. "Oral curcumin in the treatment of moderate to severe psoriasis vulgaris: A prospective clinical trial." *J Am Acad Dermatol* 2008 Apr; 58(4): 625–631.

Kurup VP and Barrios CS. "Immunomodulatory effects of curcumin in allergy." *Molecular Nutrition & Food Research,* 2008 Apr 8; 52(9) 1031–1039.

Lim GP, Chu T, Yang F, et al. "The curry spice curcumin reduces oxidative damage and amyloid pathology in an Alzheimer transgenic mouse." *J Neurosci* 2001 Nov 1; 21(21): 8370–8377.

Nagabhushan M and Bhide SV. "Curcumin as an inhibitor of cancer." *J Am Coll Nutr* 1992 Apr; 11(2): 192–198.

Nagabhushan M. Research presented at the Children with Leukaemia Conference, September 2004, www.leukaemia.org.

Natarajan C and Bright JJ. "Peroxisome proliferator-activated receptor-gamma agonists inhibit experimental allergic encephalomyelitis by blocking IL-12 production, IL-12 signaling and Th1 differentiation." *Genes Immun* 2002 Apr; 3(2): 59–70.

Natarajan C and Bright JJ. Paper presented at the Annual Experimental Biology 2002 Conference New Orleans, LA, April 23, 2002.

Nishiyama T, Mae T, Kishida H, et al. "Curcuminoids and sesquiterpenoids in turmeric (*Curcuma longa L.*) suppress an increase in blood glucose level in type 2 diabetic KK-Ay mice." *J Agric Food Chem* 2005 Feb 23; 53(4): 959–963.

Peschel D, Koerting R, Nass N. "Curcumin induces changes in expression of genes involved in cholesterol homeostasis." *J Nutr Biochem* 2007 Feb; 18(2): 113–119.

Phan TT, See P, Lee ST, et al. "Protective effects of curcumin against oxidative damage on skin cells in vitro: its implication for wound healing." *J Trauma* 2001 Nov; 51(5): 927–931.

Salh B, Assi K, Templeman V, et al. "Curcumin attenuates DNB-induced murine colitis." *Am J Physiol Gastrointest Liver Physiol* 2003 Jul; 285(1): G235–G243.

Shah BH, Nawaz Z, Pertani SA, et al. "Inhibitory effect of curcumin, a food spice from turmeric, on platelet-activating factor- and arachidonic acid-mediated platelet aggregation through inhibition of thromboxane formation and Ca2+ signa." *Biochem Pharmacol* 1999 Oct 1; 58(7): 1167–1172.

Sharma RA, Gescher AJ, Steward WP. "Curcumin: the story so far." *Eur J Cancer* 2005; 41: 1955–1968.

Soni KB and Kuttan R. "Effect of oral curcumin administration on serum peroxides and cholesterol levels in human volunteers." *Indian J Physiol Pharmacol* 1992 Oct; 36(4): 273–275.

Thamlikitkul V, Bunyapraphatsara N, Dechatiwongse T, et al. "Randomized double-blind study of *Curcuma domestica Val.* for dyspepsia." *J Med Assoc Thai* 1989; 72(11): 613–620.

Van Dau N, Ngoc Ham N, Huy Khac D, et al. "The effects of a traditional drug, turmeric (*Curcuma longa*), and placebo on the healing of duodenal ulcer." *Phytomed* 1998; 5(1): 29–34.

Wuthi-udomler M, Grisanapan W, Luanratana O, et al. "Antifungal activity of *Curcuma longa* grown in Thailand." *Southeast Asian J Trop Med Public Health* 2000; 31 (Suppl 1): 178–182.

Zhang L, Fiala M, Cashman J, et al. "Curcuminoids enhance amyloid-beta uptake by macrophages of Alzheimer's disease patients." *J Alzheimers Dis* 2006 Sep; 10(1): 1–7.

Watermelon

Alberts D, Ranger-Moore J, Einspahr J, et al. "Safety and efficacy of dose-intensive oral vitamin A in subjects with sun-damaged skin." *Clinical Cancer Research* 2004; 10: 1875–1880.

Cho E, Seddon JM, Rosner B, et al. "Prospective study of intake of fruits, vegetables, vitamins, and carotenoids and risk of age-related maculopathy." *Arch Ophthalmol* 2004 Jun; 122(6): 883–892.

Collins JK, Wu G, Perkins-Veazie P, et al. "Watermelon consumption increases plasma arginine concentration in adults." *Nutrition* 2007 Mar; 23(3): 261–266.

Edwards AJ, Vinyard BT, Wiley ER, et al. "Consumption of watermelon juice increases plasma concentrations of lycopene and beta-carotene in humans." *J Nutr* 2003 Apr; 133(4): 1043–1050.

References

Erhardt JG, Meisner C, Bode JC, et al. "Lycopene, beta-carotene, and colorectal adenomas." *Am J Clin Nutr* 2003 Dec; 78(6): 1219–1224.

Jian L, Lee AH, Binns CW. "Tea and lycopene protect against prostate cancer." *Asia Pac J Clin Nutr* 2007; 16(Suppl 1): 453–457.

Lucotti P, Setola E, Monti LD, et al. "Beneficial effects of a long-term oral L-arginine treatment added to a hypocaloric diet and exercise training program in obese, insulin-resistant type 2 diabetic patients." *Am J Physiol Endocrinol Metab* 2006 Nov; 291(5): E906–E912.

Yogurt

Anderson JJB. "Calcium, phosphorus, and human bone development." *J Nutr* 1996; 126: 1153S–1158S.

Baharav E, Mor F, Halpern M, et al. "Lactobacillus GG bacteria ameliorate arthritis in Lewis rats." *J Nutr* 2004 Aug; 134(8): 1964–1969.

Belko AZ. "Effects of exercise on riboflavin requirements of young women." *Am J Clin Nutr* 1983; 37: 509–517.

Bender DA. *Nutritional Biochemistry of the Vitamins.* New York, NY: Cambridge University Press, 1992.

Berner YN and Shike M. "Consequences of phosphate imbalance." *Ann Rev Nutr* 1988; 8: 121–148.

Beutler E. "Nutritional and metabolic aspects of glutathione." *Ann Rev Nutr* 1989; 9: 287–302.

Gill HS, Rutherfurd KJ, Cross ML. "Enhancement of immunity in the elderly by dietary supplementation with pro-biotic *Bifidobacterium lactis* HN019." *Am J Clin Nutr* 2001 Dec 74; 74(6): 833–839.

Groff JL, Gropper SS, Hunt SM. *Advanced Nutrition and Human Metabolism.* New York, NY: West Publishing Company, 1995.

Guerrant NB and O'Hara MB. "Vitamin retention in peas and lima beans after blanching, freezing, and process-ing in tin and in glass, after storage and after cooking." *Food Technol* 1953; 7: 473–477.

Gunther CW, Lyle RM, Legowski PA, et al. "Fat oxidation and its relation to serum parathyroid hormone in young women enrolled in a 1-y dairy calcium intervention." *Am J Clin Nutr* 2005 Dec; 82(6): 1228–1234.

Hanifin JM and Reed ML. "Eczema prevalence and impact working group: a population-based survey of eczema prevalence in the United States." *Dermatitis* 2007; 18(2): 82–91.

Hojo K, Ohshima T, Yashima A, et al. "Effects of yoghurt on the human oral microbiota and halitosis." Paper pre-sented at the 83rd General Session, International Association for Dental Research, Baltimore, MD, March 10, 2005.

Inoue K, Katsura E, Kariyone S. "Secondary riboflavin deficiency." *Vitamin* 1956; 10: 69.

Ivory K, Chambers SJ, Pin C, et al. "Oral delivery of *Lactobacillus casei* Shirota modifies allergen-induced immune responses in allergic rhinitis." *Clin Exp Allergy* 2008 Aug; 38(8): 1282–1289.

Jacques PF, Kalmbach R, Bagley PJ, et al. "The relationship between riboflavin and plasma total homocysteine in the Framingham Offspring cohort is influenced by folate status and the C677T transition in the methylenetetrahy-drofolate reductase." *J Nutr* 2002 Feb; 132(2): 283–288.

Perdigon G, Valdez JC, Rachid M. "Antitumor activity of yogurt: study of possible immune mechanisms." *J Dairy Res* 1998; 65(1): 129–138.

Larsson SC, Bergkvist L, Wolk A. "High fat dairy food and conjugated linoleic acid intakes in relation to colorec-tal cancer incidence in the Swedish Mammography Cohort." *Am J Clin Nutr* 2005 Oct; 82(4): 894–900.

McNulty H, McKinley MC, Wilson B, et al. "Impaired functioning of thermolabile methylenetetrahydrofolate reductase is dependent on riboflavin status: implications for riboflavin requirements." *Am J Clin Nutr* 2002 Aug; 76(2): 436–441.

Merrill AH, Lambeth JD, Edmonson DE, et al. "Formation and mode of flavoproteins." *Ann Rev Nutr* 1981; 1: 281–317.

Meurman JH. "Probiotics: do they have a role in oral medicine and dentistry?" *Eur J Oral Sci* 2005; 113: 188–196.

Meyer AL, Micksche M, Herbacek I, et al. "Daily intake of probiotic as well as conventional yogurt has a stimulating effect on cellular immunity in young healthy women." *Ann Nutr Metab* 2006; 50(3): 282–289.

Science News. "Bacteria can help lower cancer risk, University of Ulster expert says." *ScienceDaily.com* 2005 Mar 28. Available online at: www.sciencedaily.com/releases/2005/03/050325145217.htm (retrieved Oct 6, 2008).

Science News. "Is probiotic yakult helpful in the treatment of irritable bowel syndrome?" *ScienceDaily.com* 2008 Sept 12. Available online at: www.sciencedaily.com/releases/2008/09/080910090238.htm.

Villena J, Racedo S, Aguero G, et al. "*Lactobacillus casei* improves resistance to pneumococcal respiratory infection in malnourished mice." *J Nutr* 2005 Jun; 135(6): 1462–1469.

Woodcock EA, Warthesen JJ, Labuza TP. "Riboflavin photochemical degradation in pasta measured by high performance liquid chromatography." *J Food Sci* 1982; 47: 545–555.

Zemel M, Richards J, Mathis S, et al. "Dairy augmentation of total and central fat loss in obese subjects." *Int J Obesity* 2005 Jan; 29: 391–397.

Zemel MB, Thompson W, Milstead A, et al. "Calcium and dairy acceleration of weight and fat loss during energy restriction in obese adults." *Obes Res* 2004 Apr; 12(4): 582–590.

Index

About the Authors

Andi Phillips is a culinary arts instructor and recipe developer based in Los Angeles. She has headed a comprehensive elective culinary program for more than ten years, leading her students to win several scholarship awards and imparting an infectious passion for food science. Additionally, she creates recipes for *Better Nutrition* magazine, as well as for Surfas in Los Angeles, where she conducts cooking demonstrations that attract standing-room-only crowds including local chefs and food hobbyists.

Ayn Nix is editor-in-chief of *Amazing Wellness* magazine in Los Angeles. She has been writing about food and health for more than a decade for magazines including *Let's Live, American Fitness,* and *Better Nutrition.* She enjoys cooking in her spare time. This is her first book collaboration.